Yoga Storie~ ~~~~ ~~~~ Guptananda

How to be Happy and Healthy

Yoga Wisdom Explained

TESSA HILLMAN

Yoga Stories from Guru Guptananda

This book is Part 2 of an updated version of Guptananda's Stories
First published online in 2008
Second Edition (Book 1) Pub. SifiPublishing 2019
Second Edition (Book 2) Pub. Top of the Village Publishing 2022
topofthevillagepublishing.co.uk

Contact: tessa.hillman2@gmail.com
Website: yogastories.co.uk
Illustration: Alan Nisbet, Tessa Hillman
Cover design: handmade-media.co.uk

ISBN paperback: 978-1-7399846-2-5
ISBN ebook: 978-1-7399846-3-2

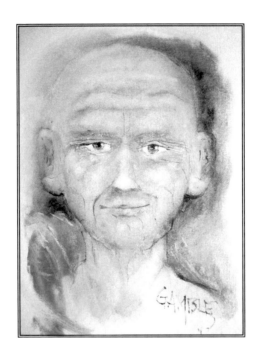

Swami Ramesh Guptananda

Portrait by Patrick Gamble, psychic artist April 2002

CONTENTS

INTRODUCTION

FOR YOUNGER READERS

Greetings all young yogis out there! I've made this book for you. You are interested in yoga, you may even have a lovely bendy teacher, but they might never tell you what the ideas behind yoga are. That would be a pity because these ideas are actually the most important part of yoga.

The stories in this book are about the life of an Indian *swami* called Ramesh Guptananda. He was a teacher of yoga philosophy — that's what *swami* means. Many funny and interesting things happened throughout his colourful life and this book features real-life stories about Guptananda and his family, to help explain different aspects of yoga.

1

In **Chapter 1**, you can find out about Guptananda, and this will help you to understand how the stories fitted together during his lifetime.

As you read, try to imagine a kind, elderly man with a gentle Indian accent is speaking to you about his life, it will add to your enjoyment of the book.

Sometimes Guptananda talks as if he is telling the story about another person, almost as if he is embarrassed to admit to some of the things he did in the past. After all, even a guru (a spiritual teacher) may not be perfect. Guptananda always takes care to admit the truth.

If you just want to read the stories, go to **Chapter 1** and read ABOUT GUPTANANDA, then skip over the grey pages to Story 1 about the first limb of yoga, and the story MY AUNT'S CHAOTIC HOUSEHOLD.

In **Chapters 2, 3,** and **4** you will find more stories about the life of Guptananda all about the **eight limbs of yoga, the three gunas,** and finally **the chakra system**. All of these make up the whole book, which you can go back to again and again as you encounter different situations and challenges in life, looking to Guptananda for wisdom.

In this book you will find the idea that there

is more to life than what we can see, hear and feel. There are many religions in the world and they are all reaching out to a Higher Power, which some people call 'God', the 'Source', the 'Great Spirit' or the 'Universe' and other names too. This book has a Hindu background and the principles in it are very similar to the Ten Commandments of the Bible. However, this book is about spirituality rather than religion.

You don't have to be religious to enjoy and learn from Guptananda's stories. They are stories to make you smile and think.

INTRODUCTION

FOR YOGA STUDENTS, TEACHERS AND PARENTS

Each chapter starts with a short explanation of the subject. The stories follow on.

We discover in **Chapter 2** the eight limbs of yoga; these are rather like the branches of a tree. Each branch is important, it has a job to do in our lives. We start at the lower branches and work our way up until we are ready to reach the top of the tree. The lowest branch is about how to conduct ourselves in the world — how to act towards ourselves and others. The next branch up is what we do with our bodies — the physical exercise.

Finally, after learning the skills of the other branches, we reach the top of the tree, fully understanding what our lives are about.

We feel happy and fulfilled...until the next challenge comes along. Then we must apply what we have learnt and overcome the difficulties in front of us. We will then find we have the tools to deal with the new problems.

Chapter 3 teaches us about the 'states of being'.

There are three states: the first is laziness or ignorance, the second is restless activity and the third is goodness and purity.

Chapter 4 explains about the energy centres, known as *chakras*. Most therapists and complementary health practitioners understand about the existence and purpose of the *chakras*, which affect us on three levels: mind, body and spirit. Many doctors in India recognise them, but in a lot of other places, such as Europe and America, the *chakras* are generally not understood. Guptananda's stories show how the *chakras* fit into our lives.

At the end of each story there is a NEW WORDS list explaining the words that come from the ancient Indian *Sanskrit* language. These words are written in italics. The list also explains less common words from the English language, to help students increase their vocabulary. All

NEW WORDS have a * next to them. The glossary at the end of the book lists all the NEW WORDS in one place.

The questions at the end of each story help readers to think about the meaning of the story and see how the story can help with understanding their own lives.

Yoga gives us a 'road map' for living. I have not covered all the different parts of yoga — there is more to learn — but I hope this book gives a good start to those beginning their yoga journey.

The Great Little Book of Yoga Stories began life online.

In Book 1, Guptananda's stories are about the Rules of Life — the code of conduct that people need to follow in order to be happy in themselves and happy with others. Book 2 also covers these, but in less detail.

Many teachers in countries where English is a second language have used these stories to help children learn about life's moral code, to learn how to be healthy in mind and body, and to improve their English, skills that will last these children a lifetime.

NOTES FOR YOGA TEACHERS

Swami Guptananda said: 'There is no point in teaching your students spiritual practices unless they are following the rules of life — the *Yamas* and *Niyamas*.' This can be difficult when your students are more mature and often many years older than you, the teacher. This is where stories come in so handy — you are not preaching, you are giving food for thought, and perhaps offering material that may be useful for their own children or grandchildren.

There are several ways to use this book.

1. Read the book yourself and meditate upon those subjects that jump out at you. Do they reflect areas in your life that could do with some attention?

2. Read some of the shorter stories to your students or to your children.
3. Choose one of the subjects at a time, and work with it for a week or a month on yourself, in your classes or with your family.
4. Précis some of the longer stories, putting them into your own words, taking care not to give the whole game away. You may give your students an appetite to read the book and benefit from it for themselves.

While this book is designed for young people who want to learn more about yoga and the stories behind it, different sections can be relevant at different ages as children mature and grow. In the section on *Bramacharya* in Chapter 2, sexual self-control is explored in a safe yet subtle manner, and the importance of the sacral *chakra* in Chapter 4 includes caution and respect when talking about sexual activities. Because of all these things and the lessons young people can learn from Guptananda's stories, this is a good book to come back to year after year as life presents different encounters and challenges.

CHAPTER 1

ABOUT GUPTANANDA

Guptananda always enjoyed helping others. Even as a small child he was deeply affected by other people's needs. He had a gentle sense of humour and a kindness about him that draws us into his stories. He didn't mind laughing at his own mistakes. This book is full of stories about his life from the age of four until his mid-twenties.

Ramesh Guptananda and his family lived very many years ago in Northern India in a comfortable house with grounds and servants' quarters. They were *Brahmins* (from the priestly class) and Guptananda's father was the chief scribe at the temple. His work was to write out and illustrate holy texts. His mother supervised the servants at home. Five servants looked after the house and grounds. Ramesh had a brother called Anil, who was born two years after him, and a sister Usha, who was four years younger than Ramesh. His family called him Ramu for short.

Ramesh was very proud to have a horse, Raja, whom he loved dearly and who features in some of the stories. At the age of sixteen, Ramesh decided to follow a spiritual path. He found a guru who was willing to take him on as a trainee monk, who he lived and travelled with for several years. In his twenties he thought that family life would suit him better. His uncle arranged a family gathering where he met a lovely girl, Meera, and they were married within a few short months. Ramesh then worked alongside his father as a scribe in the temple. After ten years of a very happy, though childless marriage, sadly, Meera died. Ramesh then decided to return to the path of the holy man, living and travelling with his guru, helping and advising people on their spiritual growth.

These tales are about family, temple and village life, providing funny or touching incidents that show us how the 'values' or 'rules of life' apply to everyday living. In this book, Guptananda explains some of the more important aspects of yoga and shows how they fit into ordinary lives.

Names of the main characters:

Ramesh Guptananda — often called **Ramu** by his family

Anil — Ramesh's brother

Usha — Ramesh's sister

Meera — Ramesh's wife

Rajendra — Ramesh's father

Mother — Ramesh's mother

Uncle Sanjay

Arun — the gardener

CHAPTER 2

THE EIGHT LIMBS OF YOGA

Younger readers might want to just skip on to the first story, on page 18, but teachers, parents and yoga students need to read this section.

THE EIGHT LIMBS OF YOGA EXPLAINED

The Eight Limbs of Yoga are different practices or skills that people can learn, in order to work towards reaching 'enlightenment'. Some say yoga is the 'Quest of the Soul'. Enlightenment could be described as a deep understanding of the meaning of life and our place in the world.

Patanjali, an ancient sage or wise man, described the eight limbs of yoga as follows:

1. *Yamas*
Controls or things we should avoid doing.

2. *Niyamas*
Self-disciplines or things we should do to be healthy and happy.

3. *Asana*
Postures and physical exercises to keep the body healthy.

4. *Pranayama*
Breath control.

5. *Pratyahara*
Withdrawal of the senses.

6. *Dharana*
Concentration.

7. *Dhyana*
Meditation.

8. *Samadhi*
Blissfulness, ecstasy.

First, we need to be living in harmony with ourselves and other people. This is where the moral code and code of conduct come in — the *Yamas* and *Niyamas* that make up the first two limbs of yoga. The *Yamas* are sometimes called controls or restraints*, because they are things we **should not** do. The *Niyamas* are self-disciplines, or 'positive duties'; they are things we **should** do.

Then we need to improve our health and energy levels by practising physical exercises, the *asanas*, and breath control, known as *pranayama*. These are the third and fourth limbs.

If we are doing our best to follow the *Yamas* and *Niyamas*, and our health is good enough for us to be able to work on our minds without the distraction of pain, we may be ready to move on. The next limb will lead to the ability to meditate. Some people who are in pain a lot actually train themselves to meditate to relieve pain.

In order to begin to meditate, first of all we have to learn to withdraw the senses from all the distractions of daily life. All the sights, sounds, smells and feelings that constantly attract our minds can be shut out temporarily when we learn *pratyahara* or sense withdrawal — the fifth limb. We don't try permanently to withdraw ourselves from what life has to offer. It is something we learn to do in order to meditate for short periods of time.

For those who have decided they want to follow the path of the monk or nun, and to devote themselves to the spiritual life, then a great deal of withdrawal from life's normal activities is involved. This book is for ordinary people living in the world in a normal way.

When external things do not distract us then we can practise *dharana* or concentration — the sixth limb.

When we can concentrate on a chosen subject like a beautiful flower or a candle flame for a certain length of time, perhaps five minutes, we find we can start to meditate. The seventh limb, *dhyana*, or meditation, can lead to a wonderful sense of being at peace. The eighth limb of yoga is a state of peacefulness or bliss known as *samadhi*.

We may consider how these eight limbs of yoga can be included in everyday life. When we follow the code of conduct we feel calm and at ease. We enjoy the company of others and they appreciate us too. This gives us confidence in ourselves. Physical exercise keeps bodies healthy and breathing exercises draw more energy into the body, so now we are healthy and energetic as well as calm and confident. The last four limbs relate to spiritual practices, which put us more in touch with our 'Higher Selves' or the 'God Force'. This brings a much deeper meaning to life and helps us through life's difficulties. Yoga is a way of living, as you will see on your journey through this book.

The eight limbs are explained in more detail in the stories that follow.

STORY 1

First Limb of Yoga
The Controls —*Yamas*

The following are the five main *Yamas*:

Non-violence — **Ahimsa**

Non-stealing — **Asteya**

Non-greed — **Aparigraha**

Truthfulness — **Satya**

Chastity or Sexual self-control — **Bramacharya**

MY AUNT'S CHAOTIC
HOUSEHOLD

When I was about twelve years old I spent some time with my Aunt Savitri and her large family. My sister Usha and I stayed with them for about a month as my mother was ill and could not look after us children. We came from a family where everything was very well regulated. My mother and father watched over us carefully. They taught us what was right and wrong. They trained us kindly but firmly. We knew where we stood.

If we disobeyed the family rules we were expected to make amends in some suitable way. For example, if we were unkind to each other we would have to do kind and helpful things and tell our parents exactly what we had done, until they thought we had done enough to make up for our unkindness.

If we shouted too loudly, or too often, we had

to spend a certain amount of time being quiet. If we were very greedy, we were given what my mother called 'second best' food to teach us a lesson. 'Second best' food was not popular in our house! It meant we would be served last of all and the food would be cold and sometimes burnt. It was the food that ordinarily would have been scraped out of the pan and used to feed the animals.

If we told lies we had to sit in a corner at mealtimes. It was very embarrassing and we were not allowed to join the family until we had felt the shame of our dishonesty.

If we ever fought or hit each other, we had to walk to the furthest well on our grounds and carry water back to the house for the servants to use. It was thought that hitting other people showed that we were too full of 'damaging energy', and that energy needed to be used up by our doing useful things.

In general, my brother and sister and I were well behaved. My parents always explained to us why we should not do this or that. The punishments I mentioned were used very few times, but just enough to remind us what was expected of us when we disobeyed our parents.

However, when we stayed at my aunt's house,

things were different. She had a large family. There were eight children and seven servants to look after them; some of the servants were children themselves. That's how it was in those days. Aunt's family was noisy, mischievous and did things that I would never have dreamed of doing.

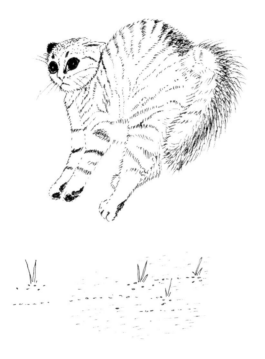

One day, three of the boys caught a cat and tied it to a tree, then started to use it for target practice. They had made peashooters and they were aiming at the cat.

When it yowled and leapt in the air, they roared with laughter. I told them that I thought they were being cruel to the cat, so they fired at me instead. When their father appeared he just laughed and said that the cat would not stay around if they treated it like that. He pointed at me and said, "As for Ramesh, he has no choice about staying here, so unless you want him to shoot at *you* with peas, you had better stop!"

I put on my fiercest face to show them that I agreed, but I started to wonder what my father would have done in the circumstances. The fact is that he would have been so shocked at such cruelty that his disapproving face would have been punishment enough. I expect he would have had us carrying water from the well for at least a week, and double the normal quantity, for being cruel to dumb animals.

My aunt and uncle's family went in for chaotic behaviour. They would shout and scream and beat each other one day and the following day all would be peace and calm, until the next incident arose.

We were having a calm day, I remember, when one of the young girls, Gopika, came and screamed at Usha and started tugging at her clothes.

"That's mine!" she shrieked. "It's my favourite dress and you've stolen it!"

This was not true at all. I recognised Usha's dress. Mother had given it to her just before we had celebrated *Divali* — the Festival of Light.

Usha burst into tears and, defending her, I said, "You are making a mistake, Gopika. This really is Usha's dress."

But Gopika would not agree. She stamped her feet and pummelled Usha with her hands. My sister flung herself at me, crying, "Ramu, she's hurting me and she's going to tear my dress!"

I looked at the others. They were all laughing harshly.

"Come on Usha," I said. "You come with me. We'll go and tell Aunt so that she can sort it out."

My aunt was not very understanding. She just shouted at us. "Of course it's not Gopika's dress," she said. "I can't afford material like that. I expect she'd like it though. You'd better sleep on it, Usha, in case she tries to take it in the night!"

I could not believe my ears. It was as though my aunt let her children do whatever they wanted. It seemed like a very disorderly way to bring up a family. One day we heard that one of the servant girls had run off with the grain merchant's son and that she was going to have a baby. My aunt was furious.

"After all I've done for her, this is what she does. She's so ungrateful!"

In truth, my aunt treated the servants badly and it was no surprise to me that the girl had run away. I couldn't wait to leave either! It was a pity the girl was expecting a baby, because she had told me she didn't like the young man very much. Although I was only twelve, I could see that she was just exchanging one difficult life for another.

The final straw came when we were all gathered together for a family celebration, an unusual event in my aunt's family. There was much squabbling and arguing over who could wear what. The menu was a source of much anger and disagreement and finally, when the day came, the servant who was the main cook fell ill. My aunt was furious; she would have to cook the food herself. She screeched her way through the preparations, making everyone feel thoroughly uncomfortable. She was not a good cook and at the end of the day, most of the dishes were either burnt or underdone. She was in a thoroughly bad mood and, to cap it all, my father turned up!

My aunt and uncle were barely polite to him

and he could sense the atmosphere, and smell the disgusting food.

"I have come to say that my wife is feeling better now and that Ramesh and Usha can return home," Father said. I am ashamed to say that I turned three cartwheels in a row, something that I have never managed to achieve before or since that day. Father whisked us away almost immediately. My sister and I could not stop grinning and holding on to Father as we walked away from that chaotic household.

"I won't ask you how it was," said Father, as soon as we were out of earshot. "I'm sorry you have had to stay so long, but it looks to me as if you have learnt a lot about how not to behave. I hope it wasn't too horrible for you. Your Aunt Savitri seems to have changed a lot since I last spent time with her. Perhaps her husband has something to do with it."

"I think you may be right, Father," I said, trying to be very grown up about it. "He's very unkind to her and to the children. In fact, they're all unkind to each other most of the time." Then I remembered a day when Aunt had sat Usha on her knee and stroked her hair when she was feeling homesick. "Aunt would be kind I think, if she didn't have so many people shouting at her."

"Everyone needs love and peace. That's what we try to provide for you at home," said Father.

"There wasn't much peace in that house," said Usha and she went on to describe what the boys had done to the cat.

My father looked shocked and then said, "So which one of you two tied the boys to a tree and shot peas at them?" We looked at him to see if he could possibly be serious. The corner of his mouth curled up, just a little, and he tousled our hair. "Neither of you? Good, I'm very glad to hear it!"

Some questions to ask yourself:

? **Non-violence** Can you think of some examples where violence was used in the story? Remember that violence can come in different ways, through thoughts, words and actions.

? Non-greed There are two sorts of greed, one is for more food than we need and the other is greed for possessions, or things we want to own. What is the example in the story of the second sort of greed?

? Non-stealing Usha's cousin wanted her dress, and was prepared to steal it. Think about stealing in as many ways as you can — there are a lot! Some sorts are worse than others. Sometimes people are forced to steal in order to survive. How should they be judged?

? Truthfulness What is the example of a person not telling the truth? How do you feel if you do not tell the truth, or if someone lies to you? Do you feel that people can still trust you, or that the person who lied is to be trusted?

? Sexual self-control — *Bramacharya* We don't know much about the servant girl who became pregnant, except that she didn't even like the father of her baby. Sometimes people make bad decisions or are persuaded to do dangerous things and have to live with the consequences. The girl would have had to bring up a child, although she was no more than a child herself. Think about it.

First Limb of Yoga

THE KUMARS AND THE CHAUDHARYS

In my village there were two notable families — notable because everyone knew them by their reputations. One family was the Kumars and the other the Chaudharys. They were well known for completely different reasons.

Let us first remember the Kumars. In Book 1 there is a story about 'Big Kumar' selling a donkey. Not only was Big Kumar a rogue*, but so were all the other members of his family. The men would cheat and lie to everyone they dealt with. They even 'double dealt' amongst themselves; no member of the Kumar family trusted any other member of that family. Their looks were guarded; their words were sly. They would prey upon strangers in the marketplace.

They were frequently in jail. They would argue and fight each other and did not hesitate to steal each other's wives. Even their children carried lines of worry and fear on their faces. Those who knew them sought to avoid them at all costs. They appeared not to understand any of the common rules of behaviour and acted more like animals than people. Everyone kept away from them except for the Chaudhary family.

The Chaudharys were a large and happy family. They had a stall at the market, as did the Kumars. They could always be trusted. They would never overcharge for the food they sold. It would always be clean and pure. They would not dream of adding sand to the salt or spices they sold. They did not try to hide old, stale vegetables beneath the fresh ones. If someone returned to their stall with a complaint, they put it right straight away. If anyone at market cut or hurt themselves, Mrs Chaudhary or one of her sisters would immediately go to their aid. Any fresh goods unsold at the end of the day would be given to the poor. They would never gossip or spread malicious* rumours about anyone. People would come and tell them their troubles and the Chaudharys would listen with a sympathetic ear; they would cheer the troubled one with a smile or a joke or a good piece of advice.

The Chaudharys were the only people who would visit members of the Kumar family while they were in jail.

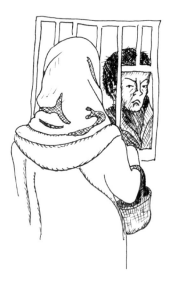

They would take food and blankets and listen to the prisoners' woes. All of the Chaudharys had open smiling faces. They loved everybody and everybody loved them. All except the Kumars, that is.

The Kumars were jealous of the Chaudharys and hated them in spite of their kindness. They couldn't understand why the Chaudharys were successful and popular while they were not.

There are no prizes for guessing which family was paying heed* to the Yamas — non-violence, non-stealing, non-greed, truthfulness, chastity — and which acted in ignorance!

> **NEW WORDS**
>
> **Malicious:** having a wish to harm
>
> **Paying heed:** to take notice of, to listen to
>
> **Rogue:** a person who is dishonest or mean

Some questions to ask yourself:

? Why might a family behave as badly as the Kumars? The Kumars show us examples of how people who do not follow 'the rules of life' might behave. Just remind yourself of that list of Yamas and think about the story.

? Does it seem as if the Kumars learn from their mistakes? They are sent to prison in order to be punished for their wrongdoings. Does that seem to be the right way to change them?

? What do you think might help them to change?

STORY 3

Second Limb of Yoga

The Self Disciplines — *Niyamas*

The following are the five main *Niyamas*:

Cleanliness — *Saucha*

Contentment — *Santosha*

Self-study — *Svadhyaya*

Self-discipline — *Tapas*

Devotion to God — *Ishvara Pranidhana*

A CHANGE OF HEART

I decided at the age of sixteen to become a monk. In my culture, this kind of decision could be changed without shame or criticism. You will find several stories about my life as a monk, including one where I was determined not to get involved with a girl. By the time I was twenty I felt I'd had enough of the life of a 'holy man'. I felt the need to settle down to family life. I returned to my family home. My mother was so delighted, she used the pet name of my childhood.

"So, Ramu, you have returned to us. I'm sure you have learnt a lot during your travels and your studies with your guru. But how will you adapt to family life now? What will you do?"

"Do not be concerned, Mother," I replied. "I am well versed in the scriptures. I can take up work in the temple alongside Father. It will not be a problem."

So my father made an opening for me in temple

life. There was plenty to do. Being a junior I had to do quite a lot of menial* work at first, but when the priests saw the quality of my script and understood fully how my experiences had matured me, I was soon given interesting and important work. I would be sent to discuss various unwritten scriptures with holy men. It would then be my job to record those meetings, to translate those words of wisdom into *Sanskrit**. Soon my mother became quite agitated, saying that I was losing my healthy glow.

"Too much writing and thinking," she said. "You need to go and spend some time on Uncle Sanjay's farm."

I agreed to go, as I had not altogether settled back into the routine of family life. It is always difficult for a young person to return to the way of life he or she had as a child. One's parents still want to advise and help, and also to control and regulate. I did not feel comfortable with this any more. I needed my freedom. Staying with Uncle Sanjay would be a good start.

There was a festival in my uncle's village. Many visitors had arrived. To my surprise I found myself sitting next to a beautiful young girl, Meera, and her family as we watched the dancing display. I felt that I wanted to know all about her. Her mother and my uncle were nodding and smiling at us, and we found ourselves free to talk uninterrupted for most of the afternoon. Suddenly I knew that this was the girl for me. Everything about her appealed to me — the way her eyes smiled, the way she paused to think before saying anything, the look of her, the smell of her — everything was right!

At the end of the day, her family were invited to my uncle's house where they stayed on for three days. During this time Meera and I got to know each other well enough for us both to know that we liked what we saw very much indeed. I found out later that my uncle had arranged this meeting, as he knew from my father that I was unsettled. He had known the girl's family for many years and had watched Meera grow up to be a very sweet and interesting young lady. He thought we would make a very good match. My parents approved and within six months we were married.

We were both very happy indeed. We lived in temple accommodation. I would work during the day at the temple. Meera would often come with me, as there was plenty of work of all sorts to be done. We were never blessed with a family although our relationship was full and complete.

I found that the discipline I had learnt as a monk stood me in good stead as a husband. Though I was disappointed not to become a father, I knew that contentment with one's lot leads to happiness, so I accepted our fate and did not lament* the lack of children. We led a well-regulated life; we worked well and played well, often walking along the riverbank, swimming and having picnics. We were self-disciplined, so we stayed healthy and happy. We had plenty of nephews and nieces to keep us amused.

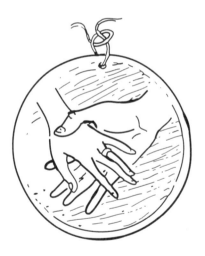

If we did argue we would give each other the opportunity to express the grievance and we would try to come to a decision that suited both of us, if possible. We tried to understand each other and ourselves and to learn from our mistakes. We did not harbour* unkind thoughts about each other or anyone else, keeping our hearts and minds as clear as we could.

All the time in the background was a recognition of our place in the world; that each of us had a soul which was part of that Great Divine Soul, or God. We would give thanks for our part in the divine nature of things. We lived a busy life full of interest and excitement, happiness and sadness, challenges, successes and some failures.

After ten years of very happy married life my wife took ill and died. I was distraught* but after a period of sadness, I came again to realise that there was still a place for me in the world. I chose to return to my life as a monk, travelling and teaching until I could carry on no longer. The *Niyamas* played a great part in my life, leading me to contentment and happiness. I found it very useful to have the guidelines mapped out by people cleverer than me. Everyone has choices to make throughout life. In the end, hopefully, each individual learns for him or herself what leads to the greatest good for all.

NEW WORDS

Distraught: anxiously worried, distracted

Harbour: to keep a thought or feeling, typically a negative one, in one's mind, especially secretly

Lament: feel sorry about or regret

Menial: work that doesn't require much skill

Sanskrit: an ancient Indian language used in all old Indian texts and writings

Some questions to ask yourself:

? Can you think of some ways in which each of the following *Niyamas* are important in your life, and why?

Cleanliness
Contentment
Self-study
Self-discipline
Devotion to God

? How could you improve on each area of your life, bearing in mind these values? If you think there are lots of things to work on, perhaps try just one for two or three weeks. It takes that amount of time for a new habit to stick. If you try to do too much at the same time you are more likely to give up and make no changes at all.

Third Limb of Yoga

Postures and Physical Exercise — *Asana*

ANIL WILL NOT ALWAYS WIN THE MATCH

This story is about me, the young Guptananda, and Anil, my brother. Anil had left the family to live on the farm with our aunt and uncle. I was the eldest in the family and my brother, who was close to me in age, had left as a young boy to keep my childless aunt and uncle company. There was a certain friendly rivalry* between my brother and myself. I missed him when he left home, but we saw each other at least once a fortnight. He chose his new life on the farm, it suited him very well. He grew fit and strong, and was proud of his muscles. Aunt and Uncle adored him and fed him very well so that he could cope with the hard work.

I was always more studious than Anil. I chose

to follow my father's line of interest and would spend a lot of time scribing passages from the holy scriptures, enjoying the perfection of the shapes of the letters and the wonderful meanings conveyed by the words. My body became fairly thin and weak and Anil gave up asking me to wrestle with him because he began to win too easily.

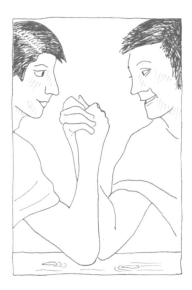

The time came when I decided to follow the teaching of a wise old man who lived five miles from us. I would go to see him regularly, usually on my horse. One day he said to me:

"This learning is all well and good, but what

is the use of a mind stuffed with information if the body is not fit to use that information?"

"I do not understand, *Swami*," I replied.

"Well, you know what it is like when someone walks into a room and you look at them and think, 'Now there's a strong person. They look as if they could cope with any difficulty!' Then someone else walks in who is weak and thin, you don't register the same impression of them. You may doubt they would be able to complete any physical test. When the strong person speaks with authority on any matter, you may be inclined to believe what they say. When the weak person speaks, you may find yourself wondering whether this person knows what they are talking about. They are not an authoritative figure, they don't appear to be in control of their body, so you may think, 'How can they be in command of their mind and are they to be trusted?' These same thoughts also occur to people when they see someone who has over-indulged and has become fat. People are more reluctant to take them seriously. But in truth these judgements are nothing more than that — judgements which people commonly make. There can be reasons of health and background that must be allowed for. Pointing a finger of blame is not the way to go, but what we can do is take control of our own lives.

"The real reason for looking after one's body, the vehicle of the soul, is to keep the body healthy and free from pain and disease. It is difficult to concentrate on our higher aspirations* if we are ill and suffering. Everyone should exercise their body adequately to keep all the muscles, joints, glands and organs working correctly. Everyone should be aware of their posture. A slumping body doesn't just make a person look unappealing, it also brings pain and tension into the muscles and joints.

"I suggest you pay more attention to your body, young man. Try walking to see me. Set off earlier. Let your horse walk beside you and ride him only when you are truly tired. Breathe deeply while you walk and walk tall. Fill your lungs with air. Bring the 'life force'* into your body. You will find that you soon become fit and you will surprise your brother in your ability to wrestle with him."

After six months of walking to see my teacher I challenged Anil to a wresting match. He won again but not without something of a struggle. He thumped me on the back and grinned from ear to ear.

"Well," he said, "all that praying and meditation can't be doing you too much harm!"

NEW WORDS

Aspirations: goals, aims or ambitions

Life force: the energy that circulates through all living things and gives vitality and strength

Rivalry: competition between people

Some questions to ask yourself:

? Have you thought about the purpose and importance of physical exercise in your life?

? How could you set about taking more care of your body, making it less likely to become unwell in times of stress or infection?

STORY 5

Fourth Limb of Yoga

Breath Control — *Pranayama*

FATHER EXPLAINS THE IMPORTANCE OF DEEP BREATHING

My family was always kept busy doing all sorts of things to keep the household going. There would be all the cooking, the preparing and of course the growing of food. There was the cleaning, both inside and outside the house, the laundering of all our clothes and the repairing and building of the house and outhouses. The horses needed to be cared for and the other animals needed to be fed, cleaned and watered. Then, we children had our studies to do. Our mother was the main supervisor of all this work.

Father worked at the temple and we would only see him early in the morning and in the evening. Sometimes he had a day off and every so often he would decide that it was time the family went on a picnic. We would always choose to walk down by the river, finding one of many pretty spots to stop at. We children would run off and play at the water's edge while Mother and Father looked on. Then my father would take off his robe and sit in his loincloth* in the shade and start doing his breathing exercises. Sometimes we would ask him what he was doing and he would motion us to go away and leave him in peace.

When we asked Mother why he was breathing like that she just said, "Your father is drawing in good things from the air. He always feels better after he has done his breathing practice. He does it every day, you know, but here by the river he has time to spend longer at his breathing exercises. Off you go and play now, we will call you when it's time to eat."

On one occasion my curiosity could not be restrained. We had all gathered round to eat our picnic. Mother was handing out large leaves filled with a delicious mix of peas, beans and tasty herbs.

I asked, "What is it in the air you like so much, Father? Can we get some too? Do we need it or are you different from us?"

"Ah, my son," said Father. "You are right to want to enjoy the benefits of breathing air deeply. Yes, you certainly can do it too, but not while you are eating, my child!" he added as I began to hold my breath with a mouthful of half-chewed beans sitting on my tongue.

"There is a wonderful thing called *prana** or life-force energy, which is in the air. The slower and deeper we breathe the more *prana* we get into our bodies. This *prana* keeps us calm; it keeps us healthy. Children get lots of *prana* into their bodies when they run around and play, when they laugh and when they shout and cry. They do all these things much more than adults do. When you get older you need to practise breathing exercises to make sure you get enough *prana*. If you do not you may become weak and ill."

"But Mother doesn't do breathing exercises, does she?" I asked.

"Many people choose not to," Father answered, "and say that if they do, they do not feel any benefit. That is up to them. I have always felt the benefit, so I will always practise *pranayama** until I become too old and weak to sit up in the sunshine."

"You'll never be that old, Father," said my sister, laughing.

"Mother says that you'll live till you're a hundred and fifty, and then you'll fly to heaven. I think you'll probably puff yourself there with your *prana* thing!"

Everyone laughed and when we had finished eating, father showed us how to make a reed pipe and blow a long string of bubbles into the water.

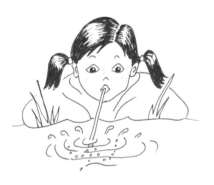

"This is how I learnt to breathe slowly," he said, as he showed us his bubbles rising one after another quite slowly in a fine stream, unlike ours which came out all of a rush, bursting the water's surface all in one go.

NEW WORDS

Loincloth: a single strip of cloth wrapped around the hips; in certain hot countries this is the only garment some men wear

Prana: a flow of energy that people can learn to sense or feel in their body

Pranayama: breath control. It is made up of two *Sanskrit* words. *Prana* means life force, or vital energy, particularly the breath. *Ayām* means to extend or draw out. So, *pranayama* means 'to extend the breath'.

Some questions:

? Have you ever tried holding your breath when you are swimming under water? You know how it feels when you run out of breath. You can train yourself to extend your breath and make it last longer. This must be done gradually over time — weeks, months and years. It is a useful skill and can help people to feel more energetic, but also more calm. Early training must be done carefully and with a teacher, as the lungs are delicate and must not be forced.

? Did you know that *pranayama* of a very simple kind helps to make us feel calm in difficult times? Try breathing deeply, in for a count of six and out for a count of six. Go on for a while. Don't force it. Stop if it feels uncomfortable. It is a useful skill for when we are feeling nervous or afraid.

STORY 6

Fifth Limb of Yoga

Withdrawal of the Senses — *Pratyahara*

RAMESH MEDITATES IN THE HAYLOFT

The story begins with me, the young monk, doing what I could to achieve 'enlightenment'*. Of course I wanted to achieve it tomorrow or even sooner... I would have long discussions with my teacher on many aspects of yoga and he would say to me, "My son, be patient, you have to take one step at a time. You cannot understand 'this' before you have fully understood 'that'."

He would often close our conversations with that statement. Sometimes progress felt very slow. I would sit in meditation and I would hear the birds singing and people working and my mind would be on them. I would want to be out in the fresh air, walking amongst the trees

52

or chatting with friends and exchanging gossip. Sometimes it was very hard to drag my mind away from all the distractions and if I tried to meditate with my eyes open, that would put an end to my meditations. There would always be something that my eyes would alight upon to remind me of the work I had not yet finished, or a person I urgently needed to see.

As an answer to such problems my teacher told me this: "To achieve 'one-pointed attention', first we must take ourselves to a place where we will not be disturbed or, if this is impossible, we must gain the co-operation of our family members so that they know when not to disturb us. Then we must make ourselves comfortable. It is difficult to meditate if pain or pressure distracts the mind.

"Having withdrawn from the sense of touch by arranging the body in a good position, sitting with back straight and hands in the lap, we must close the eyes. It takes a lot of training to meditate with eyes open. The sense of sight is so alluring* it will take the mind on a journey very readily. Then we need to observe any sounds we hear, recognise them and ignore them, thus cutting off the sense of hearing. The survival instinct will immediately bring us out of reverie* or meditation if something happens which requires us to move for our own safety's sake.

"Finally, having withdrawn most of the senses we have to hope that nobody decides to start cooking the dinner so that the sense of smell and the memory of taste are stimulated! Thus, if we withdraw our senses we are not distracted from our purpose and we can proceed with the process of concentration and on to meditation."

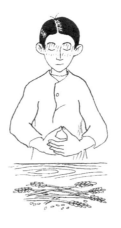

I always tried to follow my guru's advice, so I would meditate in the hayloft where no one would find me and where my body was comfortable. I could close my eyes knowing no people or animals would approach me. No cooking would be going on in the stable, so I was free from the tantalising aromas of food that might make my stomach rumble and my mouth water! The only drawback was that I would occasionally fall asleep in the hay and my family would accuse me of being lazy...

Some questions to ask yourself:

? This story is about learning to take our minds off the daily distractions of life by deliberately turning our attention away from them. What distractions can you think of that you find difficult to ignore or get away from when you are trying to concentrate on something?

? Can you think of ways to avoid those distractions while you are learning about 'withdrawal of the senses'?

? What effect does being peaceful with no distractions around have on you? Try it for ten minutes and see.

? Do you feel you need to fill your head with sounds and have people around you all the time? Meditation in a quiet and peaceful place is known to be good for both mind and body. It is a skill that can easily be learnt when you get good guidance from a teacher you trust.

Sixth Limb of Yoga

Concentration – *Dharana*

GUPTANANDA COUNTS THE BOATS

Once, when I was a young man and regularly visited my guru, I was given a task to do. My guru said to me, "Listen well, my son. Enlightenment is not for those whose minds flutter like the butterflies in the daytime, or the moths at night.. The mind must be steady and calm; the eyes must remain bright even when the lids are closed. Concentration is required in all efforts made towards achieving your goal. Occasionally you can allow yourself to daydream, yes. There will be times when the mind needs to rest, but in general you must concentrate upon your task with 'one-pointed attention'. In that way you will achieve more, and faster than most people who wander through their lives in a half dream.

"I suggest you go to the river and watch the boats as they go by. Count the number of boats with sails and the number with paddles between the time of your arrival and your departure. There won't be many sailing boats, so it shouldn't be too difficult. Do this for two hours. Come back and report to me."

I thought this was a very strange request for my guru to make of me and I could not see the connection between the number of boats on the river and my path to the Supreme One*. However I followed his instructions.

The next day I was by the river shortly after sunrise, counting the boats. It was surprisingly busy. People were getting their work done well before the heat of the day. I decided to count the boats as they passed between me and a marker on the other side of the river. I thought this would make it easier for me, preventing me from counting the same boats twice. There I sat. Two sailboats arrived that were heading in opposite directions, one upstream and one downstream, then a small rowing boat, then a canoe.

Very soon I had completely lost track of the number of boats with sails and boats with oars, so I decided just to count them all together. I added my two numbers and thought that that would have to do. Then, after a while, I realized that I had missed several boats passing because a beautiful hawk flying over the river had distracted me.

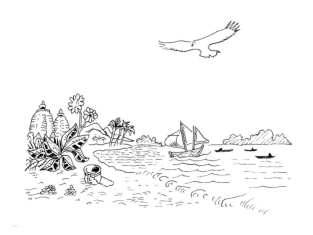

I decided to start again, this time using small stones to help me remember how many boats of each sort had passed. This pile would be sailing boats and that pile would be rowing boats. Dutifully I counted them. The sun became hotter. An ant column decided that I was in their path and they started to walk over me and up my legs. I jumped about, smacking my body where they had bitten. I scattered my stones. Which pile was which? Which were the uncounted stones and which were the 'boat piles'?

I began to get angry. I had wasted at least an hour of my time. I stomped home. In the evening I went to my guru. He seemed to know what had happened.

"Ah, my son, the birds of the air and the insects in the grass have conspired against you and turned you away from your task. How will you respond when people, who are after all much more determined than God's creatures, try to turn your mind away from your path? There is much to learn, my son, much work to do, but do not be despondent*. Here, take these counting beads. They may help you next time!"

I have to admit I glared at my teacher. "Don't worry," he said. "I won't ask you to do it again, but I think that task may have shown you something about concentration today, if only that there is a lot to be learnt!"

Despondent: low in spirits through lost hope or courage

Supreme One: God

Some questions to ask yourself:

? Are you good at concentrating on the task in hand or do you flit from one idea or activity to the next? Concentration is a skill and a discipline that you can improve on.

? Why do you think the guru gave Guptananda the task of counting the boats?

? Can you think of ways to improve your concentration?

? How important is perseverance (stickability) to being successful in achieving our aims? Can you think of a time when you persevered and were rewarded by it?

STORY 8

Seventh Limb of Yoga

Meditation — *Dhyana*

MOTHER'S QUIET TIME

In some people's minds meditation is thought to be rather strange; they think it is something done by religious fanatics and people who have cut themselves off from normal society. My story is to show you that meditation can be a part of normal life.

When I was a child and my father worked in the temple, my mother, my brother, my sister and I would be at home. Mother had several servants who helped with the work in the house and garden, and who looked after the animals. Every day Mother would have a meeting with the servants before they started their work. We children would still be in bed, but sometimes if I got up early I would see them all sitting down outside in our courtyard.

Mother would greet them all with "*Namaste*" and bow her head and they would also bow, then they would all sit in silence for a few minutes. They would close their eyes and no one would speak. The silent period would be ended with the ringing of a little bell, which my mother always had with her. It was the same bell she used to summon the servants when she needed help. Then my mother would tell each person what she wanted him or her to do that day and ask if they had anything to say. Sometimes they brought up problems they were having with some aspect of the work, but usually they would just bow and smile and thank God for their health and strength and for the gift of another new day. Thus it was in our house: everyone was peaceful and contented.

One week, however, my mother's sister came to stay. I remember Mother decided not to have the morning meditations. Her sister was about to give birth and had come to us for her confinement*. Mother told the servants what to do briefly at the beginning of each day and listened to their problems, but had no quiet period before the start of the working day. What a terrible week that was! Everyone seemed to be arguing with everyone else. Nothing was going right.

My mother forgot to buy the *dahl* (lentils) at the market, so we all had to eat nothing but *chapatis* (bread) and some tired vegetables. Mother was so preoccupied with her sister that she seemed to forget about us. This was to be my aunt's first baby so it was a very big event for her. Meanwhile my brother fell off the horse and broke his arm and my sister nearly fell down the well! Two narrow planks of wood, which had been carelessly placed over it, saved her. She was very shocked.

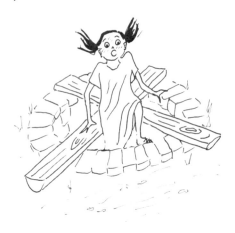

Mother blamed the servants for not covering the well properly, but I knew it had been me. I was to blame. I had been watering the animals, drawing the water up with a bucket, when Raja had bolted. I hastily threw two pieces of wood over the brickwork hole and chased after my horse.

After several days without the meditation, everyone was extremely irritable and exhausted and my father couldn't understand what had come over his family.

"Surely your sister is not so important that she can be allowed to upset all the family and servants with her new baby, which isn't even born yet?" he said.

Then my mother explained how she had stopped organising a quiet period at the beginning of the day because of being so busy.

"Ah, I see the problem now," said father. "Everyone thinks they are so busy that they have no time to sit and reflect on the day, on their work and on God's gifts. Well, you see what happens when we don't spare ourselves just a few minutes of peace? We get chaos. Surely we can find five or ten minutes at the beginning of the day to be calm and thoughtful and to ask the Lord what it is that we need to know and do each day? From now on let my family return to its previous ways and the baby will be born into an atmosphere of calmness and contentment rather than one of anger and chaos!"

The baby was born two days later and she was named *Shanti**.

NEW WORDS

Confinement: the time at the end of a pregnancy during which a woman gives birth

Shanti: peace

Some questions to ask yourself:

? Can you imagine or remember what it feels like when everyone is rushing about panicking about being late for school or to catch the bus or whatever? Think about a time when something like that has happened. What are the dangers or problems that could occur when people are in that state?

? What can we do to avoid it happening? Giving ourselves ten minutes of quiet time can help a lot, but not if it makes us late! Self-discipline will tell us to get up a bit earlier to make allowances, so we can do what we need to do in good time.

Eighth Limb of Yoga

Blissfulness, Ecstasy — *Samadhi*

THE YOUNG MONK STICKS TO HIS PLAN

After several years as a monk, I did decide to return to everyday life. However, this story happened in the earlier days of my time as a *sadhaka**. As a young man, sometimes I found the choice I had made to remain single and study ancient scriptures rather difficult to stick to. I saw my guru regularly and I travelled to different towns and villages on foot, reliant upon my good health and the generosity of other people for my food and shelter.

Even as a young monk I was called upon to perform religious rites* for people. They expected me to know all about the various ceremonies that a normal family might participate in, such as the birth of a child, betrothal* and marriage, and illness and death.

I was very happy to perform these ceremonies. I took care to look tidy and to be very clean all the time. Amongst my small collection of possessions I had a comb, a file for my nails and a toothpick. I would use certain wild plants to chew to keep my mouth feeling fresh and my teeth clean. People always appreciated and even admired my appearance and this gave me confidence to perform my religious duties, even at quite a young age. However, my looks did cause me a certain amount of difficulty.

I would find that women would react towards me in different ways. Some, usually the younger ones, were very shy and embarrassed in my presence.

With them I had to be very reserved and respectful. Others became giggly and would nudge each other and flutter their eyelashes, tilting their heads so that I could only see the lower parts of their eyes, hidden beneath their eyebrows. Towards these ladies I had to be somewhat aloof*, but also respectful of course.

Still others would try to mother me. They would advise me about matters of health and keeping warm at night and regarding my diet, what I should and should not eat. With these ladies I would quietly listen to what they had to say. I would not agree or disagree, but would merely nod my head to show that I was listening and that I had heard their advice. I think I reminded them of their sons, perhaps, but I had to maintain my position of authority, so I would not encourage their helpful counsel.

All these minor problems of human relationships would colour my days. I have not mentioned the attitude of the menfolk yet. They might be friendly, respectful, aloof, suspicious, or even slightly disdainful*. However, most of them were glad to have me around to officiate at the ceremonies for them, as hiring a priest was expensive. Since I was a wandering monk, the only payment I required was food, a roof over my head, somewhere to wash, and occasionally people would give me a new robe to replace my old one. They liked to see the monk looking his best for their ceremonies!

Now what does all this have to do with *Samadhi*? Blissfulness is a very personal thing and comes in many forms. What I have found is that when I am managing my relationships well, when my heart is neither angry or fearful, or tormented by forbidden love, I feel at peace. I am able to give good service to people and they are happy when I am at peace. I don't mind whether I sleep in a bed or on the ground, or whether my bowl is filled with plain rice or delicious fruits. Neither am I distracted by longings or desires for that which I do not have, when I am at peace.

As you may imagine, this feeling of peace and blissfulness comes and goes. For most people it is not permanent. There is much to learn in this life, many different circumstances and people to deal with, many challenges to take. I learnt that whenever I set out to achieve something new I would always feel slightly fearful about the outcome. Would I fail or would I succeed? Would I live or would I die? But I learnt not to be afraid of fear itself. If we always avoid fear then we always avoid challenges and our lives become dull and boring. We are unhappy and we don't know why. The opportunity for blissfulness is harnessed* to the courage to move on, to develop ourselves and to take our challenges willingly.

I will give you an example. After I had learnt all I needed to know about ceremonies and rites, my teacher felt I should go out into the world for a while to put some of this learning into action. I wasn't so sure. I was still a very young man and was afraid that people would not take me seriously. Not wanting to look like a complete novice, I decided not to wear my best robe. I started quite close to home in a village about ten miles away, where I thought some people might recognise me. An uncle of mine lived nearby. If all else failed I could go and stay with him.

On the day of my arrival there was a big festival going on. I was immediately drawn in to help, as there was so much to be done and not enough people who knew what to do. I have to admit I did feel quite important. I was given a good meal and a bed for the night at the house of a minor official. He was not a rich man and he told me that his daughter was betrothed* to a young man from my village, and asked if I would I conduct the wedding ceremony. The local priest had fallen ill and the marriage ceremony was due to take place the next week. I readily agreed and stayed in his house for the week before the wedding.

This man had another daughter, younger and more beautiful than the first, but the father had told her she must wait until her sister was out of the house before she would be considered as a bride.

This young girl was very lively and I felt my attention being drawn towards her. In the evenings the family would entertain themselves with music and dancing, and I was invited to be present. I felt obliged to attend, but at night it was hard for me to sleep as I kept thinking about the girl. I wondered if I had done the right thing with my life — indeed I was free to change my mind. I could marry if I wanted to and perhaps work in the temple as my father did. In fact a few years later I met and married Meera. At this point however, by morning I was certain that I was doing what I truly wanted with my life and that women had no part to play in it. However, the girl thought otherwise. She too had noticed me and started to watch my every move.

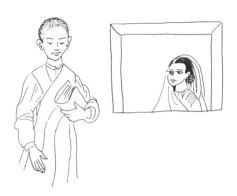

If I went to the market she would follow, and therefore I felt obliged to be with her to keep her from harm. She spoke to me of her life and told me how important temple life was to her. She would help distribute the offerings of food to the poor. She would help wash and clothe the sick. She said it would be hard for her to find a husband who shared her interests, and how she feared her father would want her to marry a merchant. I listened to her quietly.

After five days the young lady asked me why I had given up the world of family life. She thought the wandering, contemplative* life would not suit me at all. Again I slept very badly. The longings of my heart, and indeed my body, to be joined in love to this young woman were becoming fairly overwhelming. Was I to fail at the first hurdle? Was I to give up my lifetime's aim the very first time a pretty girl tried to divert my attention? I was in torment. No blissfulness at all. It was very difficult.

The day of the wedding arrived, the bride looked beautiful, but her sister more so. Then I met the groom. What a shock! I knew him from my childhood days; we had played together.

"So here you are, Ramu!" he said. "I heard you had started your new life." He looked me up and down. "This your first marriage ceremony then? Don't worry, we won't notice if you make any minor mistakes. Just don't marry me to the wrong sister, that's all. But I can see there's no chance of that, the way she looks at you; she'll have you if she can! But I know you, Ramu, you never were the marrying kind, always off studying or meditating. She's got her eye on the wrong man, hasn't she?"

I laughed, "Quite right, Gopi, there's no chance of me marrying. It's just not part of my plan." These words seemed to break the spell, on that occasion at least. I conducted the ceremony, accepted some rice and a new robe given to me to mark the occasion, in spite of my protests, and I left. That night I slept in a barn. I felt blissfully happy because I had completed my work, stuck to my plan, and I had not compromised* myself or the girl in any way. People had respected me and I had respected them. I had passed my first test.

Although this is not quite the blissfulness that comes to those who experience a feeling of deeply understanding their God, it is more like the kind of blissfulness that ordinary people experience every so often, and very wonderful it is too!

NEW WORDS

Aloof: distant, reserved

Betrothal: an engagement ceremony or event

Betrothed: engaged to be married

Compromised: risked harming someone's good name or reputation

Contemplative: thinking deeply and seriously

Disdainful: feeling or showing scorn, contempt or aloofness

Harnessed: joined to

Officiate: To conduct or carry out ceremonies

Rites: ceremonies or rituals used to celebrate certain times in life, such as birth and marriage

Sadhaka: a person who follows a particular spiritual practice or way of life

Some questions to ask yourself:

? This story is about 'blissfulness', just one aspect of it, when the person feeling blissful is perfectly content with their life at that moment in time. Can you think of a time when you have felt this?

? Do you think it is possible for human beings to be in this state permanently?

? The answer to the above question is probably no! Might you be able to explain why that is so?

? How can we achieve more blissfulness and less of the feelings we don't enjoy, like anxiety, anger or unkindness?

? Might concentration (*Dharana*) and meditation (*Dhyana*) be able to support and guide us in this?

CHAPTER 3

THE THREE *GUNAS*

THE THREE *GUNAS* EXPLAINED

The yogis say there are three ways of being, or states of existence. They are known as the three *gunas*. Most of us fluctuate* from one state to another. The idea is that we need to progress from the lowest state to the highest.

The lowest state is called *tamas*. It is a state of boredom, laziness and ignorance. It may also be described as delusion*, inertia*, apathy* and darkness. It is a low energy state of being. The kinds of food we eat can affect the state we are in. You might have heard the expression 'We are what we eat'. It means if we fuel our bodies with good healthy food we become healthy. *Tamasic* foods are stale, rotten or over-processed* and full of chemicals. These foods should be avoided. They are not satisfying and leave you feeling sickened or still hungry. When people are in the *tamasic* state they are not happy.

The next state is called *rajas*. It is a state of restless activity. A person in this state is often agitated or stressed. They may be overexcited or angry, full of lust, hatred or greed. They may be deceitful, fickle* and easily distracted, as well as ambitious and acquisitive*. Their speech may be sour and their stomach always hungry. The kinds of food that aggravate this state are sour, bitter, salty, pungent and burning. Alcohol and caffeinated drinks are considered *rajasic*. Meat eating is also known to encourage fiery passions.

The third state is *sattwa*. In this state a person is fearless and pure. They are generous and self-controlled, gentle, truthful and free from anger.

A person in the *sattwic* state is calm, happy and contented. They are able to concentrate well and achieve much. In their hearts and minds they feel serene and peaceful. The foods that help them to achieve this state are fresh, light, nourishing, juicy and soothing. Fruit, vegetables and dairy products are recommended. However, no amount of *sattwic* food will lift a person from either *tamas* or *rajas* if their attitudes have not changed first!

Sattwa has been translated as illuminating, good and pure.

It perhaps needs to be noted that *Ayurvedic*

medicine (an ancient Indian system of diagnosis and treatment), may suggest that people of certain types will benefit from eating a certain amount of sour, bitter or spicy food. These foods can have beneficial effects on some people and are not necessarily 'bad'. They are foods which are to be taken in small quantities, as it is recognised that, if the body consumes too much of them (e.g. vinegar and hot spices), it will respond badly.

NEW WORDS

Acquisitive: wanting to gather possessions

Apathy: lack of interest in things

Delusion: belief in something that is not real

Fickle: changeable or unreliable

Fluctuate: to vary, or to keep changing

Inertia: not wanting to do anything

Processed: when something is treated and changed from its natural state, as happens with processed foods

STORY 10

First *Guna*

IS BHOLA LAZY?

Uncle Sanjay had a farm. My brother spent a lot of time there and would come home with all sorts of tales about things that had happened to him during the week. He worked with Uncle from Monday to Friday and came back home at weekends. One Saturday he arrived home looking rather worried.

"What's the problem, son?" asked my father, quick to notice the frown on Anil's face. "It's Bhola, the boy who works for Uncle," said Anil. "He's making life difficult for me. I feel I am being blamed for things which Bhola has forgotten to do, or which he has done badly."

"Tell us what happened," said Father. "I'm sure Uncle Sanjay would not blame you unjustly."

"Well, last Monday my job was to milk the

cows and put them in the outdoor pen. I did as I was asked, but later on in the day the cows were found wandering up the road. Uncle thought I had not shut the gate properly, but I know I did because I remember checking it. I had not heard it click, so I clicked it hard. Then I realised it was Bhola's job to feed and water the animals and he had come in after me and left the gate open. But he did not tell Uncle that. Then on Tuesday the same thing happened again, but I was watching and I showed Bhola how to shut the gate properly. He was thankful that I explained about how it doesn't click shut properly. But on Wednesday it happened again. I was not watching and the cows got out. This time Uncle shouted at me, so I went and shouted at Bhola. He just shrugged his shoulders as if he didn't care. He did not mind if the cows wandered off and got stolen, or bitten by snakes on the wilder ground.

"On Thursday I made sure that Bhola shut the gate, then later on in the day Bhola told me that he had not fed the cattle because he could not find their food. They'd had nothing to eat all day, so their milk production was very poor that evening. Because I milk the cows Uncle blamed me again. I had to tell him about Bhola being too lazy to find the fodder for the cows, and I decided to tell him about the gate too, I was so fed up with him.

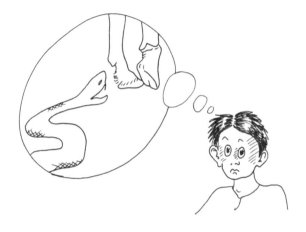

"Uncle said, 'Ah, Anil, you have always been rather impatient with Bhola. People like him need tolerance and encouragement. He is lazy, it is true, but when he does do the right thing we must acknowledge it and show appreciation. If we only ever complain to those who seem to be ruled by *tamas*, those who are slow or lazy or reluctant to make decisions, they will only get worse. When you return on Monday watch what he does right, and say something good about it to encourage him.

"'*Tamas* is a state of mind which comes from having low expectations of oneself. If other people show you that you are indeed worthy, then your mind will begin to act in a different way. If you are told you are always lazy, then you will live up to it. If on the other hand you are praised for the work you do, you will form a different opinion of yourself, and begin to live up to that good opinion.'"

"Do you agree with Uncle Sanjay, Father?" asked my brother.

"I do indeed, Anil. There was a time when it was difficult to get your brother here to clean out his horse properly. One day, after he had done it well, I pointed out to him how happy Raja was in his beautiful, sweet-smelling stall. Ramu has kept him exceptionally clean ever since. Be free with your praise and encouragement and people will respond well to it," replied my father. Being two years younger than me, Anil probably thought that I would never have been lazy; a big grin spread across his face. He turned to me, and noticed I was blushing. "Let's go and see if that horse of yours is smiling today," he said.

Some questions to ask yourself:

? There are many reasons why people might be lazy. Can you think of some?

Now think about why you too might be lazy at times.

? What would stop you from being lazy? Remember that it is very hard to change others, and that change doesn't come by willing other people to be different, but by changing our own ways of thinking and acting.

STORY 11

Second *Guna*

Restless Activity — *Rajas*

JAYANT IS NOT A NATURAL SCRIBE

There was once a family who lived in a nearby village. They were well-known to my family, as my father used to teach their son his scriptures. They would visit us each week, leave their son with us for two days and then take him back. All this was accomplished on horseback, as we had no vehicular* transport in those days.

The son's name was Jayant. He was a large gangly boy whose main interest was not the scriptures. He used to enjoy wrestling and fighting. I think his father thought a bit of scripture might calm him down a little. He was not stupid, this Jayant. He was much older than us children and he seemed almost grown up. My sister was fascinated by the beginnings of a moustache, which had started to grow on his upper lip.

On one occasion, he had come to stay with us and Father had been unable to attend to him because of some urgent business at the temple. Father asked Jayant to write out some sections of the *Vedas** and to illustrate the main paragraphs with beautiful lettering.

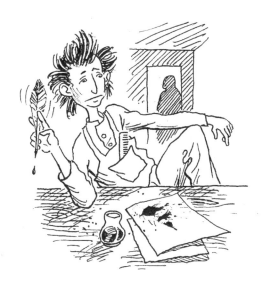

Now Jayant was not usually in the mood for illuminating letters and, on this day, nothing could have been further from what his heart desired. He yearned to gallop the horse along the riverbank, with the wind blowing in his hair, then meet up with friends, to do some wrestling, and afterwards maybe hunt some game that they could cook on a campfire on the riverbank. He told me that was what he wanted to do, and to my childish surprise that is exactly what he did! I would never dare to disobey my father like that, not at Jayant's age anyway, and I felt quite frightened for him. I remember pacing around our house and grounds, unable to concentrate on the jobs I had been given to do, worrying about what Father would say on his return. My father could be very stern at times.

The day wore on. Father returned. He asked to see Jayant, but Jayant was nowhere to be seen. "Where is the work that I asked him to complete?" asked Father, surprised at the young man's absence. "I don't think he did it, Father," said I. "Well, what *did* he do?" asked Father. "He is not here and you seem to know something about it."

I explained what Jayant had told me and to my astonishment Father's face broke into a huge smile.

"Ah, my son," said he, "young Jayant has a restless, active soul. He finds it very difficult to be calm, to sit still, to contemplate. His mind and heart are always churning, always wanting to move about, never at peace. He is ruled by *rajas**. He finds it almost impossible to quieten himself. I am surprised he has returned to work and study with me as many times as he has. I think his father made a mistake sending him to me.

"The young man's energies need to be directed into something more suitable for him. He should be training horses, delivering important news to neighbouring towns, or anything that would usefully occupy his restless body and mind. I think I shall have to tell his father that he is wasting his time and money bringing Jayant to me. This young man needs to cool down a great deal before his mind will be fit for more *sattwic** activities."

And with that Father ruffled my hair and went off to find Mother.

Some questions to ask yourself:

? It is important to choose work that suits our interests and personalities. How might you describe Jayant's personality?

? How might you describe your own personality? People can change with time. How would you like to change, if at all?

? As we get older we begin to see how different people are, and how we compare to them. Is it better to try to work with our own interests, talents and abilities and develop them, rather than copying someone else, or trying to be what someone else wants us to be? What might happen if we copy or please others all the time? How might that make us feel about ourselves?

STORY 12

Goodness and Purity — *Sattwa*

A GOOD WAY TO START THE DAY

My mother always used to start the day with a certain prayer. She said it put her in the right frame of mind, and she taught us that prayer. When I was very small I did not understand it, but as I grew I began to realise the implications of its meaning.

The prayer went like this:

"Lord*, today I awake to the beauty of the world. I glory in the sunshine and enjoy the rain. May all that I do this day be like the sunshine and the rain. May all that I do enhance* the lives of those around me and glorify your holy name."

That was the prayer. It was simple and at the same time complex. I did not understand the words 'glory' and 'glorify', I thought it had something to do with shining, so it did not make sense to me. However, one day I thought to ask Mother what it meant.

She replied: "Each day when I wake up I look at the sky and I know that the sun will shine, bringing us warmth and light. It will help the plants to grow; they are our food and our shelter. It will bring light into dark places. Then I remember that if we only had sun and no rain we would shrivel and die, so I thank God for the rain that comes in its dark and heavy clouds. I then talk about glorifying the Lord. That means that I wish to show my appreciation and thanks for all that He has given to us. When I do this each day it helps me to remember that everything that comes to us each day is the Lord's work.

"Every person who asks for help, every problem that comes along to teach us a lesson, every joy, every sorrow, all these things come from the Lord. All the love that I receive from my family and friends, and all the difficulties I have to overcome, all come from the Lord. He sends these things to help us to learn on our pathway through life. If I can bear this in mind throughout the day, then I am likely to appreciate truly all the wonderful gifts that surround me.

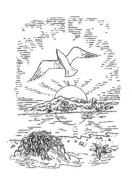

"Also, I am able to look on problems as challenges and ways of learning, rather than as burdens that I grudgingly* bear. So I live my life looking forward to whatever the Lord brings me. Many people live in dread of the next difficulty that may arise and do not notice the beauty and joy in the world around them. Instead they just fret* about the future.

"That is my prayer, Ramu, and a prayer for you might go like this if you don't like the words 'glory' and 'glorify'.

"'Dear Lord, I thank you for this day and all the gifts it brings. I will do my best to serve you and learn from the lessons you send me. I will enjoy the blessings of the sun and the rain, the plants and the animals, my family and friends.'

"If you repeat this prayer, Ramu, you will feel calm and happy and everything you do will be sincere and from the heart. Your actions and thoughts will be ruled by *Sattwa* and will be brightened by the Light of the Lord."

Some questions to ask yourself:

? Some people believe in God and the afterlife, others do not. If you do, then your ideas will be about the god of your culture. The ideas in this book can be helpful to people of any culture.

? How might a person who has no belief in any god be positive about their life? What useful thoughts can they have on waking up to a new day? Being thankful for what we do have is helpful. The way we behave towards our family and friends, and to people and animals in general, makes a big difference to the way we feel about ourselves.

CHAPTER 4

THE *CHAKRA* SYSTEM

THE *CHAKRA* SYSTEM EXPLAINED

The *chakras* are part of the energy system in the human body. Rather like the electric circuits in a car, human beings have their own energy-flow system. This is separate from the nervous system that conducts electricity around the body along the nerves. Many forms of Eastern medical practice recognise and work on the *chakra* system, and on the meridians or lines of energy, which flow around the body. You may have heard of acupuncture and shiatsu, or some other forms of 'energy treatment' that are becoming more common in the West today.

Chakras are like whirlpools of energy, which flow into and out of the body at certain points. There are many of these *chakras* or energy centres, but the seven main ones are by far the biggest and most important. These are the ones we will be learning about. The word *chakra* means wheel and comes from the *Sanskrit* language.

In the pictures you see the names and positions of these seven main energy centres.

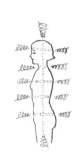

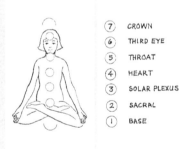

7 CROWN
6 THIRD EYE
5 THROAT
4 HEART
3 SOLAR PLEXUS
2 SACRAL
1 BASE

Our health and emotions affect the amount of energy flowing into and out of the *chakras*. The better our *chakras* are working, the better our health and our feelings about life.

They allow energy in to and out of the body. When they are working well we say they are balanced, our body is healthy and we are feeling happy. Then one of life's difficulties arises, for example one of our parents becomes ill, or we have a serious argument with a friend. These sorts of things affect our *chakras*. They can shut down or block the energy that should be flowing through them. Sometimes they become overactive and produce too much energy. Either way we start to feel uncomfortable and this feeling is a symptom of our *chakras* being 'unbalanced'.

Normally we solve these sorts of difficulties by taking a positive attitude, by talking to parents or helpful friends and by engaging in physical activities. Yoga is particularly helpful, as many of the exercises move and stretch the spine a lot. The main current of energy in the body flows up and down the spine; this current is supplied by the *chakras*. We find that yoga exercises make us feel better both mentally and physically. This positive approach helps to get the *chakras* back into balance again. If, however, we can't seem to sort out a particular problem, our energy centres may remain unbalanced. Our health may eventually be affected.

Eventually people learn to see things differently

and perhaps give up their anger or their fear, which are the kinds of emotions that unbalance the energy in the body. Counselling can be useful to help us deal with really difficult issues. Life is largely about learning to live happily with others and learning to deal with our emotions in a healthy way. There may be times when we just need to step away from people who are bad for us.

The *chakras* affect us on all levels: physical — the state of the body; mental and emotional — the state of the mind; and spiritual — the state of the soul.

We will now look at the individual chakras to discover how they affect us in our everyday lives.

THE BASE *CHAKRA* — *MULADHARA*

The first or base *chakra* is situated at the base of the spine. It is also known as the 'root *chakra*'. Its *Sanskrit* name is the *muladhara chakra*.

The base *chakra* sends its energy in to and out of the main 'river' of energy, called the *susumna*, which flows up and down the spine. From here it flows to the whole body, as does the energy from all the *chakras*.

When this centre is working well it gives us feelings of being energetic, active and lively. Our survival instincts and also the desire to have children (the instinct to reproduce) come from this centre. When we are well connected through this centre we feel 'grounded in reality', rather than living life in a dream world. The story illustrating the base *chakra* is about survival.

STORY 13

The Base *Chakra*

TRAVELLER'S TALES

In the old days, when I was about twelve years of age, if I remember correctly, we were going on a journey, my father, mother, brother and myself. This was quite an unusual occurrence for my family. We were going to see my father's eldest brother, my old uncle. He was unwell and not likely to live much longer. A messenger had come to bring us news of him. Father decided we should all go and Raja, my horse, could do the carrying. The journey would take two days and we had to take food and water to last us. We would stop overnight in one of the villages along the route and stay with my aunt when we arrived.

When at last everything had been gathered and packed, and then repacked by my mother — who said father had no idea how to pack belongings, especially his own — we set off. It was before dawn. We had to travel in the cooler part of the day and rest when it became too hot. As we walked along, smelling the air and listening to the waking sounds of the birds, my father told us about a journey he had made as a boy.

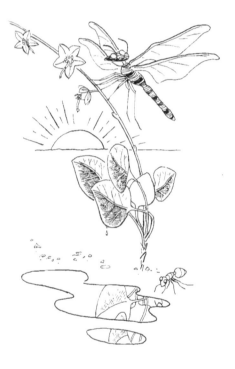

He said that thieves had set upon the travelling party. He calmed our anxious looks by saying that life had been much harder in those days and that many poor people had been obliged to rob and steal for their survival. These times were better, robbers had not been heard of for at least thirty years in these parts.

He told us how the thieves had taken everything, the mules, the horses, the food, and even the water. It had been a very dangerous situation. "I was just a lad of ten," my father explained. "I cried bitterly, but my mother comforted me saying:

"'This is bad, it is true, but do not fear. We always try to do our best for each other and for the Lord Krishna*. Let us pray to him and surely he will look after us. Let us ask him for water and food, since that is all we truly need to survive. At least our lives have not been taken away from us.

"So we all stood facing the sun," my father went on, "and asked God for his help and succour* in our time of trouble. Then we continued our journey. A lone horseman who was a water carrier* passed us after an hour or so and gave us enough water to last until the next settlement. There we made contact with some people who knew my uncle and who held him in very high regard. They furnished us with all we needed for the rest of the journey.

"We were very glad to be of assistance to their family later on in the year, when their daughter needed to stay in our village. So we all survived, with God's grace, but it's a strange feeling to have your life apparently in danger. You realise how strongly you want to cling to it and how much you love Earth and all that dwells on it."

My father entertained us with several more stories on our thankfully uneventful journey. I was relieved to arrive at my uncle's village safely, nevertheless, and I was even more relieved to get back home at the end of our little adventure.

NEW WORDS

Lord Krishna: the Hindu god Vishnu is said to have become a man called Lord Krishna on Earth thousands of years ago

Succour: help or relief given in time of need

Water carrier: a *bhisti* was a person who carried water in animal skins from wells to a where it was needed

Some questions to ask yourself:

❓ This story is about survival and how strong a need it is for all people. What emotions might you feel if you thought you were in danger? Think of the positive emotions as well as the negative ones.

Yoga practice helps you to keep calm and not panic. Which of the skills of the eight limbs of yoga would be useful if you were feeling very nervous or afraid? Not sure? Look back at the fourth limb, *pranayama*, breath control, on page 46. If we can keep calm we make better, safer decisions.

THE SACRAL *CHAKRA* — *SVADHISTHANA*

The second energy centre is the sacral or *svadhisthana chakra*. It sits just below the navel and is named after the sacrum, a big flattish bone at the bottom of the spine. It is the main centre of joyfulness and sensuality, or appreciation of the senses. We use this centre when we are creative; creating works of art such as paintings, sculptures, models, pottery or anything that involves using our hands to make beautiful, interesting or useful things.

This is the *chakra* through which we enjoy another human being in sexual love, so it is also creative in the sense of creating babies. When we feel sexual desire and love for someone, we may become aware of a feeling of energy and excitement in this area of the body. For this energy to be used in a healthy way it should be coupled with love and respect for the other person.

We need to be very aware that our actions have consequences. This centre can produce much delight, but also much pain and suffering when used thoughtlessly, or abused. Careless sex can result in unwanted pregnancy, fatherless children, abortion and sexually transmitted diseases*.

Young people need to be educated about the dangers of this new energy that comes to them in their teenage years, or sometimes earlier. They need to use wisdom and courage to do what is best for them and avoid being persuaded to do things that they know to be unwise.

The story about the sacral *chakra* is rather old-fashioned in the sense that today's young people, in the West at least, expect to go out together as boyfriend and girlfriend. They are trusted to act responsibly, but may find their freedom confusing.

There is a lot of very poor information on the internet that can give young people the wrong idea of what to expect from their partner. The internet can be a bad influence and lead to disrespect and confusion between people.

NEW WORDS

Sacral: the area of the large triangular bone at the base of the spine.

Sexually transmitted disease: when a man or woman has a sexual disease and then has sex with a new partner, they can give or transmit that disease to the other person. They may not even know they have the disease. This is a big subject that young people need to learn about and understand, but this book is not the place for such information. Ask a trusted adult, or a nurse, doctor or teacher to help you to find information.

STORY 14

The Sacral *Chakra*

HOW A YOUNG MAN AVOIDED ROMANCE

Once upon a time, there was a young man. He might have been me, Guptananda. This young man was filled with all the sensations of a young male animal in spring. He felt an inner jauntiness*, which makes young men seek the company of young women and not just for their friendship.

He had been brought up very carefully and properly by his father and mother. He knew what he should do and what he should not with regard to young women. He knew full well that one thing leads to another, a look to a sigh to a touch and so on, and he did not feel ready for commitment. So, in general, he simply avoided looking. On this occasion, however, it was a beautiful spring day, not too hot, and he was free for the whole day. He wanted to go off and explore, but he had a yearning in his heart for company.

Walking down the road and wondering how to satisfy his yearnings, he encountered Tara, a black-eyed beauty whom he had known for many years. Now Tara also happened to be free on this day, so the pair decided to spend it together somewhere along the riverbank. Tara had always admired our friend, but he had never taken much notice of her. He had always thought her rather brash*. Not his sort at all really, but she was funny and witty and would provide a listening ear for his verbal meanderings*.

As they walked along, he saw a different look in her eye, a look that seemed to grow in intensity, a look of adoration and longing that was being directed at him. It kindled a fire within him, which made it quite difficult to follow his train of thought. After a while he fell silent and the two of them continued along the path. Every so often their hands brushed together and he felt a tingling sensation rush through his whole body. This was strong stuff, this was a heady brew*, but in the back of his mind he knew that he did not even like the girl very much. He heard his father's voice saying to him: "Do not waste your energies on women you do not love. It can lead to much pain and suffering."

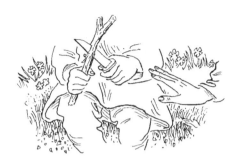

He broke a branch from an overhanging bough and, as they sat watching the river running by, she laughed and joked and fluttered her eyelashes at him, while he whittled at the wood, making a beautifully decorated piece. Finally she tired of her chatter and he, having turned his sacral stirrings into a different form of creativity, produced a gift for his mother on his return home.

His mother looked at him quizzically* as he handed the wood to her. "But what shall I use it for?" said she.

"Just wave it at me on my free days and I will remember how to spend them productively and without regret!" replied the thoughtful youth.

NEW WORDS

Brash: rudely self-assertive; bold; impudent

Heady brew: any alcoholic drink that makes people feel light-headed

Jauntiness: liveliness, carefree confidence

Meandering: wandering in speech without a goal or direction

Quizzically: questioning in a puzzled way

Some questions to ask yourself:

This story is about one of the functions of the sacral energy centre. This energy has a proper place in relationships where there is real commitment and respect between partners.

? What did Ramesh Guptananda really think of the girl?

The story shows how we can be attracted to people who are unsuitable for us. What do you think of Ramesh's behaviour on this occasion?

? If Ramesh had decided to ask her to be his girlfriend, would either of them have been happy?

THE SOLAR-PLEXUS
CHAKRA – MANIPURA

The third *chakra* is known as the *manipura chakra* in *Sanskrit*. It is situated above the navel and below the ribcage. It has several jobs to do. It is the main collector and distributor of power in the body. Sometimes this *chakra* is called the 'mind centre' as it plays a part in memory and learning. It is concerned with our willpower and courage. People with strong solar-plexus energy have a powerful and confident presence. They also have a good attitude towards keeping themselves healthy. They look after themselves.

If we are lacking in confidence and are weak-willed, not bothering to care for our bodies and eating a bad diet, we will not have a healthy supply of solar-plexus energy. If we do not get enough sleep or exercise, or if we take drugs, or drink more than a very modest amount of alcohol, then our solar-plexus energy will be low. The effect of this is that we will find it hard to summon the enthusiasm to enjoy our lives, and our bodies start to complain and become sick.

As we grow up, gradually we learn from adults how to look after ourselves. The process of growing up involves learning to take responsibility for our own actions and behaviour. Not all adults are good role models. We can learn to recognise both good and bad examples, and if we choose to follow the good ones and learn what not to do from the bad ones, then we are more likely to be happy and confident.

In the story about the solar-plexus *chakra*, Ramesh finds that he is somewhat lacking in willpower when it comes to dealing with the market stallholder. It teaches him an important lesson.

STORY 15

The Solar-Plexus *Chakra*

THE APPEAL OF A LITTLE GOAT KID

One day, when I was a boy of about fourteen years of age, my mother gave me a job to do. I had to go in to town and purchase some meat. The problem was it would all be on the hoof: live poultry, sheep and goats. I had to come back with a leg of either a sheep or a goat. I had been to market before with Mother and had watched her select an animal. It would then be slaughtered and people would draw lots* for the various parts of the carcass or, if they were determined to purchase a particular cut, they would have to pay a higher price for it.

It was important to get to market very early in the morning to accomplish this task, as meat becomes rank and foul very quickly in the heat of the day. The animal had to be killed, butchered and brought home to keep it cool in a very short space of time, or it would start to smell horrible. We had a special basket for carrying meat. We would line it with fine grass to absorb the blood and after the purchase was brought home the grass would be burnt.

So off I went to market in some trepidation*. I never liked to look into the eyes of the animals that my mother chose to be killed and I certainly did not want to look into the eyes of the animal on whose fate I was to decide! Many people were vegetarian, including my father, but the rest of my family were not and, indeed, I have to say that I did enjoy the taste of meat. On this day, however, I began to consider becoming a vegetarian.

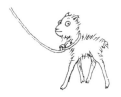

When I arrived at market there were only two animals to be seen. One was an old ewe, the other a beautiful little kid goat. I knew my family would not appreciate any of the meat from the mangy* sheep. My eyes travelled over the little goat who was standing with its back towards me. I was hoping it would not look at me as I decided its fate.

The stallholder could read my mind. He knew that he could persuade me not just to take and pay for part of the animal, but to take the whole kid, live, if he made the right moves. It was his will against mine. He was determined to get me to take a good look at the little animal and I was determined not to. He even picked the kid up, held it in his arms and stroked its little head.

"Look at him," the stallholder said. "He can't be any more than six weeks old. Why don't you take him home and, if your family don't want to slaughter him, you can keep him as a pet. He'll eat anything. Mind your shoes. He'll eat them!"

At this point, I had still managed to avoid looking at the kid's face. I kept looking over the shoulder of the butcher and sideways at the other stalls. I knew that if the goat caught my eye, that would be that.

"I want a leg," said I. "Better make it two, since he's so small."

"Which legs?" the stallholder asked. And as I looked down to show him, the kid raised his head and bleated plaintively*. I saw his beautiful eyes and his lovely face.

"I'll take all of them," I said. "Have you got any rope?" The old man winked and tied a length of rope around the kid's neck. I handed over the sum required and we walked home, the goat and I, the redundant* meat basket over my arm. My little sister met us as we neared the house. She was delighted with the kid and named him straight away. He was to be called Babu. My mother guessed what had happened immediately. She threw up her hands in feigned* anger.

"Ramu, I see you don't have the stomach for being the executioner. Never mind, there's plenty of dahl in the sack. Lentils it will be tonight. Maybe your father's brother will take Babu. He's certainly very pretty. He would make a good mate for their little goat."

Babu did indeed become a beautiful billy goat and I became a vegetarian. My courage and willpower had deserted me on that occasion and I decided never to put myself in such a position again. If I was not prepared to eat meat, I could not be asked to be a party* to its slaughter. My family understood my situation and never again told me to go to market on such an errand.

Some questions to ask yourself:

? Why do you think Ramesh was feeling nervous about going to buy the meat?

? Are you a meat eater?

? How do you think you would feel if you had to do the same job as Ramesh?

Vegetarianism is a complicated topic that we can't fully discuss here. If you are interested, be sure to find out more before making any decision to change how you eat.

Although Ramesh failed to buy the meat, his solar plexus or power centre was working well, it helped him to make a big decision: if he could not choose to kill animals, he would not eat their meat any more.

THE HEART *CHAKRA* – *ANAHATA*

The fourth *chakra,* known as the heart centre, is called the *anahata chakra* in *Sanskrit.* It is the centre through which we feel love, and is situated in the middle of the chest. Feelings of warmth, compassion and appreciation of other people come from this centre. Our love for our family, friends, pets, animals and nature in general, begin in this centre.

Sometimes, if you are with someone you love deeply, you may feel your heart centre becoming active, opening up to that person. It is a wonderful feeling. You may experience the same feeling towards a baby brother or sister, a member of your family who you don't see as much as you would like, or even towards a much-loved pet. It's a feeling of great warmth and attraction. It makes you want to hug the person or pet.

When we lose someone we love we may feel a terrible heaviness in the centre of the chest. This is how the heart *chakra* feels when it has closed down. This is the way it reacts to loss of love. Normally, as time passes, we get over our loss and it opens up again. Then we are able to love others without fear of losing them too.

When the heart *chakra* is working well we are normally happy and harmonious in our relationships with other people.

STORY 16

The Heart *Chakra*

GUPTANANDA'S DAYS OFF

When I was a young man I had a beautiful horse, Raja. I have mentioned him before. Now Raja and I used to love roaming the countryside on our special days off, when no work was required of me. Those days were few and far between, but when they were granted to me, or should I say to us, we truly appreciated them. We would ride for miles, sometimes towards the mountains, sometimes along the riverbank. My heart used to feel as if it would burst, it was so full of love for the beauty of nature, and Raja seemed to feel the same. He would trot with his head held high and his nostrils wide, taking in all the aromas around us.

He loved to go to new places. It always made him excited and especially attentive. He never stumbled on an unseen boulder. He would never walk under a branch that would be dangerous for me. As I saw him avoiding these things, I felt a rush of love for him flowing from my heart and when this happened, he would always cock his head in recognition of my emotion, as if to say, "I love you, too!"

When we returned home, my young sister would run to meet us and ask eagerly to hear all about the journey and the new places we had seen. Then I would feel my heart warm towards her too.

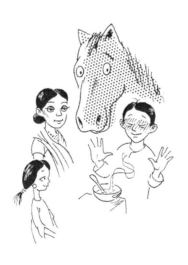

My mother would smile indulgently* and place a bowl of delicious vegetable stew in front of me, waiting patiently to hear of my travelling and at that moment, my heart would warm to her too. Then at night, before sleeping, I would give thanks to Lord Krishna for all that I had beheld that day. Once again a warm glow would fill the centre of my chest, the glow of love in the heart centre.

A question to ask yourself:

? Do you recognise the feelings described in this story? It is good to become aware of our feelings, to be able to recognise and name both the good ones and the bad. Then we can gradually become more in charge of our feelings and our relationships.

THE THROAT *CHAKRA* – *VISHUDDHA*

The fifth or throat *chakra, known as the vishuddha chakra* in *Sanskrit,* is situated in the middle of the neck. It governs the mouth, tongue and neck, and is related to self-expression and communication. When it is working well you can speak your inner truth freely and without fear. When it is out of balance, you have difficulty staying true to yourself, expressing your needs, desires and opinions to yourself or to others. Wise parents allow their child to speak and then give approval and encouragement, or guidance when needed. The old idea that 'children should be seen and not heard' would have been very bad for the development of children's throat *chakras*!

The throat *chakra* is involved in our choice of career and our satisfaction with our work, where we express ourselves in the world.

STORY 17

The Throat *Chakra*

THE TOY HORSE

This story is about using the voice. I could tell you about the time when I addressed large crowds of people, after I had mastered my throat energy, and no longer felt nervous about speaking in public. However I think the time that comes to mind and, which is more amusing, was when I was very young.

One day when I was a very small boy, my brother and I were arguing over a toy. The problem was that it was his favourite, and my favourite too. Because I was the elder, I normally got my way. On this occasion, however, my brother was determined to win the battle. The toy was a little wooden horse that my father had made for us. On giving it to us, he had made the mistake of not declaring one of us to be the true owner.

Small children are very possessive and like to

know what is their very own property. My father learnt a lesson from this experience, but to him it seemed too late to decide who was to be the owner of the horse. He thought that we could learn to share the toy. Some days we did exactly that and took turns to play with it quite amicably*. But on this day things were different. My brother was expressing his rage that I insisted on keeping the horse from him because as he said, he had an 'important game' to play. I shouted back at him that since he had had the horse for the whole of the previous day, it should be my turn today.

My father looked at both of us and, taking the horse from me, he said, "He who shouts loudest is not necessarily the right one. He who is willing to share and take turns is the right one. Since you two cannot agree to share, you are both wrong and since you are both shouting very loudly, you are doubly in the wrong. I myself would like to have a go with the horse. Why not? I made it. I am not shouting, so I am right. I am willing to take turns, so I am right again; it is going to be my turn to play with the horse today. Now let me hear you say sorry for making such a rumpus* and let us play properly."

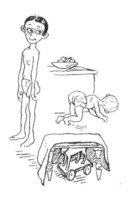

Then he invented a game where he hid the horse and we had to find it. Each time we found it we would all laugh and shriek with glee and he would point to his throat and say, "Now that's what I like to hear, happy sounds, not angry sounds."

He was a very wise man.

NEW WORDS

Amicably: in a friendly way

Rumpus: a noisy disturbance

Some thoughts:

? Have you ever felt as if you had 'a lump in your throat'? Think about when it happened. Something upsetting usually causes that feeling. The throat energy slows down and we feel blocked. It can become hard to speak.

If children are constantly told to 'shut up', or people laugh at what we say, our throat *chakra* can react. Be careful how you treat others, be kind in speech, and mean what you say with your heart — you will be looking after your own *chakras* as well as other people's if you do that.

Think about times when you have heard people talking very loudly, making other people listen to them without consideration. That might be a sign of an overactive, therefore imbalanced, throat *chakra*. The *chakras* can become overactive as well as underactive, and what people need is balance. This is an interesting subject and you might wish to follow it up in your own studies.

THE THIRD EYE
– AJNA CHAKRA

This *chakra* sits in the middle of the forehead between the eyebrows. It is the sixth energy centre, known as the *Ajna Chakra* in *Sanskrit*. This is a very mysterious centre to many from the West who have no belief or understanding of psychic* abilities, such as clairvoyance*. This centre is responsible for our intuition. When we get a very strong feeling of something that proves to be true, then it could be our intuition or third eye that is telling us this.

The third eye is involved in work of higher creativity, such as composing music, writing poetry or literature, inventing things and creating exquisite works of art. Sometimes during meditation we may see visions with our inner eye. These are often answers to questions or problems we may be having.

The Third eye

MEDITATION IN
THE HAYLOFT

One day when the young Guptananda was well into his second year of study under his guru, he was given a question. The question was this — how much time should he spend meditating each day in order to achieve a good rate of progress?

His guru would not advise him on this. He wanted the student to discover the answer. The young man was rather puzzled, because he thought that this was the sort of thing his guru should be telling him, not asking him. However, on his long walk home our friend had time to ponder on this question.

He asked himself, "What is the purpose of meditation?"

He told himself, "We meditate in order to quieten the mind and to contact the god within, who has all the answers."

"Ah," thought he, "then I will ask my god within for the answer to this one."

Some days he would sit and try to still his mind for meditation, but all the time images of his life's activities would float across the mirror of his mind. On other occasions he would fall asleep as soon as he had settled himself and he would wake with a jolt when his head touched his chest. An occurrence, which he looked forward to with a gentle, warm anticipation*, was the feeling of being in communication with another mind greater than his. This happened at times when he was at his most tranquil* and when he was in a good, receptive learning mode. He looked on this as his guidance, not sure if he was feeling the presence of God, or of some sort of spirit helper counselling him and helping him along.

On this occasion, when he reached home, the young Guptananda went straight to the hayloft where he could be alone. Only his horse moved quietly on the straw and cobbles while he perched in the rafters of the loft on a little platform he had made for the purpose. He made himself comfortable and peaceful. Then he opened his mind to the Almighty One. He asked of the Supreme Spirit an answer to his question.

He sat and waited and, as he waited, he felt a coolness on his forehead. With his eyes closed, he saw the blue starry heavens open up to him; he felt himself floating amongst those stars; and he felt as large, or as small, as any one of those stars. A great sense of peace came over him. There he stayed enveloped in peace and with the Almighty. He felt energy radiating from his limbs and his head, and finally the 'knowing' or hearing of some words:

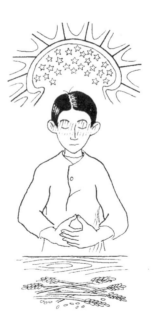

"Keep practising meditation but do not allow it to take over your life. A young man has work to do, gifts to appreciate, life to live. It is not the amount of time that matters, but the quality of openness to God."

Finally, the young man descended from the loft feeling uplifted and energised by this knowledge and power that he had experienced. He knew fully now that it had not been just his imagination at work on those other occasions when he had experienced 'meditational happenings'*. It had been real.

Guidance is at hand for whoever seeks it and whenever it is sought. His guru had explained that sometimes we are not ready for an answer. We must be content to learn at a pace that is appropriate for our own development.

NEW WORDS

Anticipation: looking forward to something

Meditational happenings: occasionally when people meditate, they may have visions, they may receive a helpful message or hear music. They may feel energy moving around both inside and outside their bodies. Sometimes people see swirling or steady colours and lights. Occasionally guides or angels appear in the mind's eye. They bring a sense of understanding and peace.

Receptive: open to receiving information or ideas

Tranquil: peaceful

Some questions and answers:

? **Can you just learn to meditate for yourself?**

It is best to have a teacher to begin with.

? What can you expect from meditation?

With a bit of practice you can expect a feeling

of peace, quiet and calmness, which affects how you feel for the rest of the day.

❓ How much time should you spend meditating?

Start with a few minutes and work up to ten minutes, any more than that and you may be wasting your time. You cannot force your mind to be peaceful. There are times when it is better to be getting on with things rather than hoping and praying for answers to come.

THE CROWN *CHAKRA* — *SAHASRARA*

The crown *chakra* is situated at the top of the head. It acts like a funnel for Universal energy to flow into a person's body. In people who are spiritually awake and familiar with the idea of having a soul and being connected to the 'Source', the crown *chakra* will be open and receiving energy efficiently.

Those who have no such beliefs or who are fearful about them may have much reduced crown *chakra* activity. They will get their energy supply from all the other *chakras* which take over the function of the crown *chakra*.

STORY 19

The Crown *Chakra*

THE GLOWING *SWAMI*

When I had been a *sanyasin* (a monk who has taken vows of renunciation*) for several years, after my wife's death, and I had travelled around my country and to Tibet, I came across a wise old man, a hermit. He welcomed me and asked if I would like to stay with him for a time. I liked the look of his eyes, the sound of his voice and the meanings of the words he spoke. This man was called *Swami* Madhusudana Vedanta. I chose to stay with him. He was about sixty-five, but as he had lost most of his hair and most of his teeth, he looked much older. One could tell from his vigour, however, that he had not yet passed into real old age.

He would meditate with me each day before sunrise and then we would walk into the nearby town to beg for food. The people always gave us enough to survive on, not a lot, but enough.

In return we would perform acts of healing* for them.

One day a woman brought us a bowl of meal. With her was her young son, a small child of about eight years of age. She was very concerned about him. He was lethargic and had a nasty skin condition on his legs. She asked 'Swamiji*' to heal the boy by prayer and meditation. She asked me to lay my hands on him, because she had heard that people had been cured by my touch. She said that the healing heat from my hands and the will of God would surely cure her son.

We agreed, Swamiji and I, to try to help the boy. Swamiji sat down cross-legged with his arms outstretched towards the boy and he started to chant. Much to my surprise I noticed, while I was resting my hands on the child's shoulders and feeling energy flow through me, that Swamiji had developed a beautiful radiance. It was particularly concentrated around his head, a beautiful golden glow.

The mother and son were apparently oblivious to this. After a while Swamiji stopped his chanting and I removed my hands from the boy's shoulders. Swamiji's head continued to glow for some minutes after he had finished. The boy raised his head and opened his eyes wide.

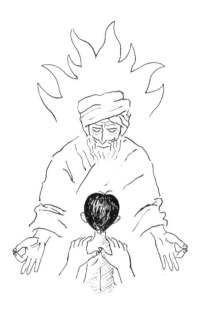

"Mama," he said, "these *swamis* are on fire. I felt it, but it was a good fire, not like when I burnt myself on the hot cinders. Yes, look, you can see the flames at the top of the old one's head!"

The mother smiled and hugged her child. Thanking us, she said, "Come, my son, the Lord Krishna has visited you through these good men. You will be better now." They then departed.

Swamiji, still sitting, raised his hands up to the heavens and then, bowing very low, he gave thanks to God.

Some questions and answers:

? Why might people go to healers?

They usually go because they can get no help from their health service for various reasons. Some go because there is no health service available to them, or they cannot afford to pay for treatment. Many people go because they feel that their problem may be emotional and possibly spiritual, and they want to seek help from a healer rather than a doctor.

If you have access to a doctor you should see what they have to say about your complaint or illness. There might well be a quick and simple solution.

Not all people who call themselves healers are genuine. You need to check on their reputation, and if they are charging large sums of money, avoid them.

? Where does the healing come from, if it happens?

It is believed to come from 'God', or the 'Universe', or the 'Source'. The healer is just a channel for the healing energy to flow through.

? Do you have to believe in God or the Universe for healing to work on you?

No, but you need to be open to the possibility that it might work, and it might change your way of thinking if it does. Healing may come in the form of a sense of calmness, a new understanding, an improvement in the health condition, and sometimes a complete cure.

You may have a greater understanding of yoga philosophy now that you have read the stories. If you read the parts of the book in grey, you will find further explanation. However Swami Ramesh Guptananda hoped that people would enjoy his stories and learn from them. For young people the stories and questions may be enough in themselves.

If you have enjoyed the book do let me know! You might like to write a review or a recommendation. Please spread the word to your yoga-loving friends. Profits from the book go to children's charities.

My website is:
　yogastories.co.uk or;
　yogastories.wordpress.com
　email : tessa.hillman2@gmail.com

GLOSSARY

This is the complete list of all the words in the NEW WORDS sections.

Please note that some words have several meanings. I have only included the meaning for the words as they are used in this book.

Aloof: distant, reserved

Alluring: very appealing

Anticipation: Looking forward to something

Be party to: to be involved

Betrothal: an engagement ceremony or event

Betrothed: engaged to be married

Brash: rudely self-assertive; bold; impudent

Compassion: kindness, understanding

Confinement: the time at the end of a pregnancy during which a woman gives birth

Contemplative: thinking deeply and seriously

Controls, or restraints: things we should avoid, or hold back from, e.g. avoid being violent or stealing

Craft: boats of any kind

Delusion: belief in something that is not real

Despondent: low in spirits through lost hope or courage

Disdainful: feeling or showing scorn, contempt or aloofness

Distraught: anxiously worried, distracted

Draw lots: to decide who will do something by, for example, choosing straws of different hidden lengths — the person with the longest straw wins

Enhance: to improve or add to

Feigned: pretended

Fluctuate: to vary or to keep changing

Fret: to feel troubled or worried

Godhead: God Almighty

Grudgingly: reluctantly or unwillingly

Guru: A spiritual teacher

Harbour: to keep a thought or feeling, typically a negative one, in one's mind, especially secretly

Harnessed: joined to

Healing: many spiritual people from all beliefs and backgrounds have the 'gift of healing', helping to make people better in mind, body and spirit

Indulgently: warmly, generously

Inertia: not wanting to do anything

Jauntiness: liveliness, carefree confidence

Lament: feel sorry about or regret

Loincloth: a single strip of cloth wrapped around the hips: in certain hot countries this is the only garment some men wear

Lord Krishna: the god Vishnu, to whom many Hindus pray, is said to have become a man called Lord Krishna on Earth thousands of years ago

Malicious: having a wish to harm

Mangy: shabby, diseased

Meanderings: wandering in speech without a goal or direction

Meditational happenings: occasionally when people meditate, they may have visions, receive a helpful message or hear music. They may feel energy moving around both inside and outside their bodies. Sometimes people see swirling or steady colours and lights. Occasionally guides or angels appear in the mind's eye. They bring a sense of understanding and peace.

Menial: describing work that doesn't require much skill

Paying heed: to take notice of, to listen to

Plaintively: sadly, wanting pity

Prana: a flow of energy that people can learn to sense or feel in the body

Pranayama: breath control. It is made up of two *Sanskrit* words. *Prana* means life force, or vital energy, particularly the breath. *Ayām* means to extend or draw out. So, *pranayama* means 'to extend the breath'.

Processed: when something is treated and changed from its natural state, as happens with processed foods

Quizzically: questioning in a puzzled way

Rajas: a state of restless activity

Redundant: not needed

Renounced: given up

Renunciation: giving up worldly pleasures

Reverie: a daydream

Rites: ceremonies or rituals used to celebrate certain times in life, such as birth and marriage

Rogue: a person who is dishonest or mean

Rumpus: a noisy disturbance

Sacral: the area of the large triangular bone at the base of the spine. The sacral area extends forwards to the lower belly

Sadhaka: a person who follows a particular spiritual practice or way of life

Sanskrit: an ancient Indian language used in all old Indian texts and writings

Sattwic: fearless, pure, calm, happy and contented

Sexually transmitted disease: when a man or woman has a sexual disease and then has sex with a new partner, they can give or transmit that disease to the other person. They may not even know they have the disease. This is a big subject that young people need to learn about and understand, but this book is not the place for such information. Ask a trusted adult, or a nurse, doctor or teacher to help you to find information on this.

Shanti: peace

Succour: help or relief given in time of need

Supreme One: God Almighty, the most high

Swami: teacher of yoga philosophy

Swamiji: a respectful way of addressing spiritual teachers in India

Tranquil: peaceful

Trepidation: anxiety or dread

Vedas: sacred books of the Hindu religion

Vicinity: an area near or around a place

ABOUT THE WRITER AND THE BOOK

This book came to me as an answer to a prayer. It had taken me three years to train as a yoga teacher, and I had been teaching for fifteen years, but I felt there was still a lot more to learn, if I was going to be able to keep teaching my students. I couldn't turn to the internet, because it didn't exist in those days. Instead, I decided to ask for help through meditation. That's how an India guru came into my mind.

He told me: "There is no point in teaching people about spiritual matters unless they are following the *Yamas* and *Niyamas* [the rules of life]."

I had to admit that although I had learned the rules when I had studied to be a teacher, I could not remember them all.

The guru became stern. "You should know the *Yamas* and *Niyamas*, you are a yoga teacher!" he said. Then he changed his manner and showed himself to be kind and patient. "Never mind, don't worry, I'll help you," he said.

On that day, in the Launceston Leisure Centre in the UK, much to my surprise and amazement, the guru gave me a little story about greed. It was from his own life and told how, as a small child, he had learnt about sharing food from his father. It was as if the guru was dictating the story to me! I had my pen and notebook so I wrote it down as he spoke.

I was about forty-five at the time and hadn't written any stories since I'd been at school. Before taking up yoga I had been a biology teacher. Nothing was further from my mind than writing stories.

Wondering if I had imagined the whole thing, I asked for another story, on a different rule of life — non-violence.

It was like the first story: quirky, light-hearted, but making a point. I found that each time I asked for a story, one came. No planning or thought was involved at all. I just needed to be fresh and alert and in the right frame of mind for meditation.

Soon I had ten stories, all about the main *Yamas* and *Niyamas*. I used them to help teach my students.

I asked my teacher what he was called, and the name Ramesh Guptananda formed in my mind. Then, when I discovered from reading about yoga that there were ten more *Yamas* and *Niyamas*, I asked for stories on those subjects, and they came.

Then life got in the way of story writing. I had a smallholding and six yoga and fitness classes and a family to attend to. But over several years, normally during the winter I managed to collect the eight limbs stories. I went on to ask Guptananda for stories to illustrate the energy centres, or *chakras*. Finally, I asked for stories on the three *gunas*, or states of being.

After that, in 2008, I created an online book containing all forty-three stories Guptananda had told me. Technology has moved on now, and my online book was no longer working perfectly. I have converted to paperback and ebooks so that my readers can have their very own copies.

Twenty odd years after meeting the guru I checked on the meaning of 'Guptananda'- Gupta means hidden and ananda means bliss, Hidden

Bliss — very appropriate! I am aware that I have promoted 'Swami Ramesh Guptananda' to 'Guru Guptananda'. I hope he doesn't mind. I feel his wisdom is worthy of a guru.

After writing the Guptananda series I found that if I meditated and asked for stories on different subjects, for example on forgiveness or being grateful, I would be given them from all over the world. I did not choose where the story should come from, but the different guides came forward to tell me their stories. They came from far and wide: from China, Australia, Russia, America, Africa, India, France, Alaska to name just a few. I collected nineteen stories about the Laws of Life of the Native American people too — maybe another book to come?

I created an educational stories blog, yogastories.co.uk in order to offer my stories to the world, and today they are used by people from many English-speaking nations, and by teachers from all over the world who need simple stories in English to help their students learn the language. Nearly half a million people have visited my stories blog.

If you have enjoyed 'Yoga Stories from Guru Guptananda' please spread the word, and look out for 'The Great Little Book of Yoga Stories' on Amazon. My next book will be about the strange happenings in my life that turned me from a total sceptic into a believer in the afterlife.

ACKNOWLEDGEMENTS

First of all, I would like to thank Gerry Hillman, my husband at the time, for his support, tolerance and patience over the several years it took to create this book.

I have also received help and encouragement from my editors Philip Jewell, Brian Davis, Carole Alderman, Jean Reynolds, Rosie Barratt and Renu Gidoomal, all of whom looked carefully through the book and suggested adjustments according to their own expertise and background. Helen Greathead, Rebecca Halkes and Chris Short edited the second Edition (Book 2) pub. 2022. Thanks to Bek Pickard for text layout and Mick Clough of handmade-media.co.uk for the cover design.

Dr Shastry, the late Academic Director of the Bhavan Institute of Indian Culture in London, taught *Sanskrit* and Hindu philosophy. He checked the book both for accuracy with regard to the Indian way of life and for its interpretation of Hindu philosophy and *Sanskrit*.

B.K.S. Iyengar, through his books *Light on Yoga* and *Light on the Yoga Sutras of Patanjali*, has been a very important source of information for me throughout my thirty years as a yoga teacher. I would like to express my appreciation of his work.

I would also like to thank Patrick Gamble, psychic artist. I asked him for a picture of my spirit guide. Patrick, knowing nothing at all about me, 'saw' Guptananda and painted a beautiful portrait of him.

My dear friend the late Alan Nisbet deserves many thanks. His wonderful illustrations enliven the book greatly. I have made a few illustrations myself, to complete the book.

I would like to include in my thanks my husband, David Guiterman, a scientist to the core, who is quietly intrigued by what I am writing. He was very skeptical, but now recognizes that there are probably other realms of existence.

This book would never have happened at all had not *Swami* Ramesh Guptananda come into my mind and given me the stories, for which I am eternally grateful.

REVIEWS

'This book is not only great for children but will also refresh and inspire adult students and teachers of yoga alike.

Underpinning the philosophy of yoga, Patanjali's Yoga Sutras and The Bhagavad Gita are interpreted and presented here in a way that makes them easy to understand and apply to our own lives, whether we are young or old.

For any yoga teacher, this book will enhance and enrich your studies and help you share these teachings with children and adults.'

Emma Mansfield, yoga teacher
and community organiser

'This book is just gorgeous and perfect right now as I embark on my children's yoga teacher journey. It provides a lovely uncomplicated way of introducing yogic philosophy into our yoga classes and will definitely spark my imagination to help me make my classes fun.'

Wendy McCartney, Kundalini yoga teacher

'Book 2 guides the younger reader through the 'Eight Limbs of Yoga'. Simple, charming and moral stories based around Guptananda's family life as a boy growing into a man, reveal how the different limbs relate to every aspect of life. Making right decisions, caring for the body and learning how to breathe correctly aids the focusing and stilling of the mind, leading to bliss in meditation. Explanations of the Gunas or 'ways of being' are given, and also examples of how our energies are influenced by the Chakra System help us learn about the interconnectedness of everything in the universe. Useful guidance for teachers is also included, encouraging deeper thinking, promoting mindfulness, reminding us that yoga is the art of skilful living.'

Sandra Chatten, yoga teacher
with 45 years' teaching experience

'It is always difficult when you are trying to explain patterns of behaviour to young people and trying to find the right way to get them to start thinking for themselves and applying what they have learnt to their own lives. Tell them and they may well reject your advice, but offer them a story and let them draw their own conclusions which are neither right nor wrong and you will help them become more rounded individuals. This book does just that. It is non-judgmental but gives ideas and room for [young people] to develop and explore emotions and behaviours in a safe environment.'

Kathy Wallis, retired teacher,
Cornish bard and storyteller

'I really enjoyed these stories and I love that they can be also used for teaching classes… I'm relatively young, so I don't want to seem as if I'm giving older people instructions on how to live. These are lovely to guide people. The questions at the end of each story are a brilliant way to allow you to reflect; bullet journaling for mindfulness is so popular now! It is a great book for introducing the lessons from real yoga (not just the postures that are usually associated with it) and invites anyone to read about it. The 'New Words' asterisks are a really nice touch for younger readers.'

Skye Talen, yoga teacher

'The stories contained within are lovely, easy to

read and suitable for everyone. The insight into the different chakras is captivating; and the morals within the stories can be relatable to circumstances encountered throughout the course of everyday life.'

Emily Morley, meditator

'This is a very delightful insight into [inner peace,] attainable through the proper working of a well-attuned mind and spirit! Reading it has been a most 'calming, settling experience' – and [a] most enjoyable 'learning' one too!'

Christopher Short, unfamiliar with yoga

'I really enjoyed reading this book, I couldn't put it down, and that's very unusual for me. I feel I know a lot more about yoga now and it was fascinating to find out through these lovely stories. I had no idea there was so much else in yoga behind the exercises and the breathing. I will certainly get a copy for my grandchildren.'

Carolyn Hindley, meditator